Brow Lift

Editor

JAMES E. ZINS

CLINICS IN PLASTIC SURGERY

www.plasticsurgery.theclinics.com

July 2022 • Volume 49 • Number 3

ELSEVIER

1600 John F. Kennedy Boulevard • Suite 1800 • Philadelphia, Pennsylvania, 19103-2899

http://www.theclinics.com

CLINICS IN PLASTIC SURGERY Volume 49, Number 3
July 2022 ISSN 0094-1298, ISBN-13: 978-0-323-84934-0

Editor: Stacy Eastman
Developmental Editor: Jessica Nicole B. Cañaberal

Clinics in Plastic Surgery (ISSN 0094-1298) is published quarterly by Elsevier Inc., 360 Park Avenue South, New York, NY 10010-1710. Months of issue are January, April, July, and October. Business and Editorial Offices: 1600 John F. Kennedy Blvd., Suite 1800, Philadelphia, PA 19103-2899. Periodicals postage paid at New York, NY and additional mailing offices. Subscription prices are $548.00 per year for US individuals, $1234.00 per year for US institutions, $100.00 per year for US students and residents, $613.00 per year for Canadian individuals, $1,259.00 per year for Canadian institutions, $682.00 per year for international individuals, $1,259.00 per year for international institutions, $100.00 per year for Canadian and $305.00 per year for international students/residents. To receive student/resident rate, orders must be accompanied by name of affiliated institution, date of term, and the *signature* of program/residency coordinator on institution letterhead. Orders will be billed at individual rate until proof of status is received. Foreign air speed delivery is included in all *Clinics* subscription prices. All prices are subject to change without notice. **POSTMASTER:** Send address changes to *Clinics in Plastic Surgery*, Elsevier Health Sciences Division, Subscription Customer Service, 3251 Riverport Lane, Maryland Heights, MO 63043. **Customer Service: 1-800-654-2452 (US and Canada). From outside of the United States and Canada, call 314-447-8871. Fax: 314-447-8029. E-mail: JournalsCustomerService-usa@elsevier.com (for print support); JournalsOnline-Support-usa@elsevier.com (for online support).**

Reprints. For copies of 100 or more of articles in this publication, please contact the Commercial Reprints Department, Elsevier Inc., 360 Park Avenue South, New York, New York 10010-1710. Tel.: +1-212-633-3874; Fax: +1-212-633-3820; E-mail: reprints@elsevier.com.

Clinics in Plastic Surgery is covered in *Current Contents, EMBASE/Excerpta Medica, Science Citation Index, MEDLINE/ PubMed (Index Medicus), ASCA,* and *ISI/BIOMED.*

Contributors

EDITOR

JAMES E. ZINS, MD, FACS
Head, Section of Cosmetic Surgery,
Department of Plastic Surgery, Emeritus Chair,
Department of Plastic Surgery, Cleveland
Clinic, Cleveland, Ohio, USA

AUTHORS

FABIOLA AGUILERA, MD
Plastic Surgery Resident, Division of Plastic
Surgery, The University of Alabama at
Birmingham, Birmingham, Alabama, USA

MOHAMMED S. ALGHOUL, MD, FACS
Private Practice, Abdali Hospital, Abdali
Boulevard, Amman, Jordan; Adjunct Assistant
Professor, Division of Plastic and
Reconstructive Surgery, Northwestern
University Feinberg School of Medicine, Illinois,
Chicago, USA

CAGRI CAKMAKOGLU, MD
Resident in Plastic Surgery, Cleveland Clinic,
Cleveland, Ohio, USA

IRENE A. CHANG, BA
Medical Student, Case Western Reserve
School of Medicine Health Education Campus,
Cleveland, Ohio, USA

MALCOLM P. CHELLIAH, MD, MBA
Department of Dermatology, Cleveland Clinic
Foundation, Cleveland, Ohio, USA

JOSHUA M. COHEN, MD
Hansjörg Wyss Department of Plastic Surgery,
NYU Langone Health, New York, New York,
USA

DEMETRIUS M. COOMBS, MD
Senior Resident, Department of Plastic
Surgery, Cleveland Clinic, Cleveland, Ohio,
USA

JAMES WALTER DUTTON Jr, MD
Aesthetic Surgery Fellow, Cleveland Clinic
Department of Plastic Surgery, Cleveland,
Ohio, USA

JAMES C. GROTTING, MD
Clinical Professor, Division of Plastic Surgery,
The University of Alabama at Birmingham,
Grotting Plastic Surgery, Birmingham,
Alabama, USA

JACOB GROW, MD
Southern Indiana Aesthetic and Plastic
Surgery, Indiana, USA

CATHERINE J. HWANG, MD, FACS
Staff, Cleveland Clinic Foundation, Cole Eye
Institute, Cleveland, Ohio, USA

SHILPI KHETARPAL, MD
Associate Professor, Department of
Dermatology, Cleveland Clinic Foundation,
Cleveland, Ohio, USA

ALAN MATARASSO, MD
Clinical Professor of Surgery, Northwell Health
System/Hofstra University, Donald and
Barbara Zucker School of Medicine at Hofstra/
Northwell, Manhattan Eye, Ear and Throat
Hospital, New York, New York, USA

ABIGAIL MEYERS, BS
Medical Student, Case Western Reserve
School of Medicine, Cleveland, Ohio, USA

JULIAN D. PERRY, MD
Staff, Cleveland Clinic Foundation, Cole Eye
Institute, Cleveland, Ohio, USA

IRA L. SAVETSKY, MD
Private Practice, Plano, Texas, USA

ELBERT E. VACA, MD
Private Practice, Boca Raton, Florida, USA

JAMES E. ZINS, MD, FACS
Head, Section of Cosmetic Surgery,
Department of Plastic Surgery, Emeritus Chair,
Department of Plastic Surgery, Cleveland
Clinic, Cleveland, Ohio, USA

Contents

rejuvenation, the mainstay of treatment of the eyebrow is operative intervention. The senior author's technique has developed over many years, first focusing on the open coronal and anterior hairline approach to the forehead lift, then the endoscopic brow lift, and most recently, the lateral subcutaneous temporal lift. This technique allows for reliable and safe elevation of the lateral brow with minimal complications.

 Video content accompanies this article at http://www.plasticsurgery.theclinics.com.

Subcutaneous undermining for brow lifting is not a new technique, but the gliding brow lift is evolutionary in the sense that it can be done through 1 or 2 tiny incisions and the brow shape maintained with transcutaneous running sutures (the hemostatic net). Undermining over the frontalis muscle and galea is performed using blunt dissectors and the lifting is done with superior traction, holding the brow in the desired shape with the hemostatic net.

Brow lifting, when indicated, can significantly improve upper eyelid aesthetics. Brow lifting is a powerful maneuver to shape and lateralize the curvature of the brow arc and directly influences the upper eyelid fold height and the curvature of the upper eyelid crease. This article reviews the importance of upper periorbital aesthetic assessment because it lays the foundation to tailor the appropriate operative intervention. Highlighted are the authors' preferred approach to aesthetically shape the brow along with other complimentary upper eyelid aesthetic procedures including upper blepharoplasty, blepharoptosis repair, fat grafting, and upper periorbital fat shifting to optimize brow lifting outcomes.

Aging of the face is a continuous and dynamic process that occurs due to changes in layers including skin, muscle, fat, and bone. There is an increasing patient preference toward nonsurgical techniques and procedures that require minimal downtime in all aspects of cosmetic surgery. The mainstay of treatment involves the administration of injectable fillers for temple volumization, eyebrow reshaping and forehead contouring, and neuromodulation to reduce the appearance of dynamic rhytids. Surgical and nonsurgical procedures can be used in combination in order to maximize periorbital rejuvenation. This article focuses on nonsurgical rejuvenation of the brow and periorbital complex.

Direct browlifting comprises various techniques to lift the brows using incisions on or around the brows. The classic direct browlift involves removing an ellipse of skin and subcutaneous tissue within or just above the brow cilia. Brow lifting techniques can be modified to address only lateral brow ptosis, modifying the incision to the mid-forehead or the eyelid crease, and placing the incisions in different areas during bilateral surgery to improve symmetry. Careful attention to incision location, closure technique, and use of postoperative therapies can allow for nearly invisible scars.

An Algorithm for Correction of the Aging Upper Face

James E. Zins and Abigail Meyers

As the approach to the upper face has evolved in recent years, so has the focus of aesthetic brow procedures. Brow position was the primary focus early in the late twentieth century, with the coronal brow lift the primary means of surgical correction. In more recent years, improving or maintaining brow shape has taken on greater importance and has increasingly been addressed by contemporary techniques. These include the endoscopic, temporal, direct, gliding approaches as well as nonsurgical brow lifts. As each patient has individual facial characteristics and expectations, every technique comes with a unique set of indications.

CLINICS IN PLASTIC SURGERY

SERIES OF RELATED INTEREST

Facial Plastic Surgery Clinics
https://www.facialplastic.theclinics.com/
Otolaryngologic Clinics
https://www.oto.theclinics.com/

THE CLINICS ARE AVAILABLE ONLINE!
Access your subscription at:
www.theclinics.com

Preface
More Than a Brow Lift: The Importance of Brow Shape

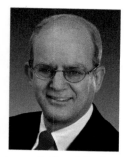

James E. Zins, MD, FACS
Editor

Very often authors writing in our peer-review journals highlight their favorite procedure. They may or may not compare and contrast their findings with the current literature. While Continuing Medical Education articles attempt to provide a full review of the literature, space constraints often make this a difficult task. In this issue, we have attempted to address the wide gamut of current surgical options with regard to the correction of the aging upper face. Using this approach, we believe that this issue is of value to the practicing plastic surgeon as well as to those of lesser experience.

The brow lift has perhaps changed more in the past generation than any other facial aesthetic procedure. The coronal brow lift, the workhorse of the past generation, has largely been replaced by a variety of less-invasive but effective techniques, and the coronal lift is rarely performed today.

The strength of an issue compiled by multiple contributors resides with the quality and surgical talents of the authors. We were fortunate to have been able to include our first-choice authors, who provided their articles in a timely fashion. For this, we are deeply appreciative.

The issue begins with a discussion of the pertinent surgical anatomy, highlighting both anatomic principles and surgical correlation. This is followed by a series of articles detailing the wide variety of surgical procedures available for the correction of brow ptosis today.

The endoscopic brow lift is described in detail and is accompanied by video illustration depicting the technique in detail. Indications and relative contraindications are clearly outlined. The hairline brow lift is included because it has undergone a resurgence due to the recent popularity of facial feminization surgery. Video illustration of the technique, including details such as means of hairline lowering, is also provided.

Success in brow lifting is no longer predicated merely on brow elevation. Perhaps the name of the operation is obsolete and should be changed from brow lifting to brow shaping. The recent importance of maintaining or improving brow shape is emphasized in Dr Mohammed Alghoul's excellent article on brow and eyelid aesthetics.

Several authors emphasize the principle that the action in brow elevation is in the subcutaneous plane. The following two articles highlight this evolving concept. The subcutaneous temporal lift highlights lateral brow elevation and is beautifully illustrated by Dr Alan Matarasso. This is followed by the gliding brow lift, an extension of Auersvald's hemostatic net. This is reviewed and illustrated in detail by Dr James Grotting. He provides a number of before and after photographs documenting the efficacy of this new and exciting technique.

Clin Plastic Surg 49 (2022) ix–x
https://doi.org/10.1016/j.cps.2022.03.003
0094-1298/22/© 2022 Published by Elsevier Inc.

plasticsurgery.theclinics.com

Dr Julian Perry and Catherine Hwang illustrate the direct brow lift and its potential for wider application. Dr Shilpi Khetarpal describes noninvasive means of improving aesthetics of the upper third of the aging face, including the use of botulinum toxin, fillers, lasers, radiofrequency devices, and microfocused ultrasound. Finally, the issue is summarized in an article illustrating our algorithm for brow lifting.

If this issue is perused cover to cover, the reader will have an updated and full appreciation of contemporary techniques for treating the aging upper face. It is hoped that this will then be implemented into his or her armamentarium of surgical techniques and result in improved patient care.

James E. Zins, MD, FACS
Section of Cosmetic Surgery
Department of Plastic Surgery
Cleveland Clinic
Desk A 60
9500 Euclid Avenue
Cleveland, OH 44195, USA

E-mail address:
Zinsj@ccf.org

Brow Anatomy and Aesthetics of the Upper Face

James E. Zins, MD, FACS[a],*, Jacob Grow, MD[b], Cagri Cakmakoglu, MD[c]

KEYWORDS

- Brow anatomy • Brow esthetics • Brow lift • Forehead lift

KEY POINTS

- An understanding of the three-dimensional anatomy of the forehead is critical to safe and effective esthetic surgery of the upper face.
- The complex anatomy of the forehead is three-dimensionally similar to the temporal region.
- The deep branch of the supraorbital nerve is easily injured in brow surgery, and understanding the anatomy will minimize this risk.
- Improving or maintaining brow shape is perhaps more important than brow lifting.

INTRODUCTION

Effective treatment of facial aging should use a global approach addressing the upper, mid, and lower face as well as the neck. In this monograph, we focus on only one of these critical areas, the upper face. When patients consult the plastic surgeon regarding periorbital aging, the focus is often on the eyelid area only in spite of the fact that the brow represents a critical part of the aging problem. It is therefore incumbent upon the plastic surgeon to raise the issue of brow rejuvenation. Often with aging, the patient loses the natural appearance of the superior orbital rim. Brow surgery can restore that loss of definition of the superior lateral orbit, whereas upper lid surgery alone cannot.

The surgical correction of brow ptosis has perhaps changed more than any other area of facial esthetics. We currently have both surgical and nonsurgical options available which now go far beyond what can be accomplished by the classic coronal brow lift. This includes the endoscopic approach, the isolated temporal lift, the direct brow lift, the transpalpebral corrugator resection, the gliding brow lift, and the chemical lift. Finally, the anatomy of this area is complex. To best serve our patients, to provide the best results, and to minimize complications, an in-depth understanding of this anatomy is critical. Although controversies exist regarding the most effective methods for brow lift surgery, a thorough understanding of the complex anatomy in this area is the foundation for both surgical and nonsurgical correction of brow ptosis.

BROW ESTHETICS

At the lowest border of the forehead, the brow marks a natural transition point from the upper to middle horizontal third of the face. The ideal position of the brow varies not only by gender but also between cultures. Iatrogenic manipulation of brow shape with makeup, manual hair removal, and the more recent utilization of microblade tattooing are common. Just as trends exist in clothing fashion and hairstyle, what could be considered an attractive brow has also undergone evolution over time. While still appreciating this variability, anatomic tenants of brow

[a] Section of Cosmetic Surgery, Department of Plastic Surgery, Cleveland Clinic, 9500 Euclid Avenue, Cleveland, OH 44195, USA; [b] Southern Indiana Aesthetic and Plastic Surgery, 2450 NorthPark, Suite B, Columbus, Indiana 47203, USA; [c] Cleveland Clinic Department of Plastic Surgery, 9500 Eucllid Avenue, Cleveland Ohio 44195, USA
* Corresponding author:
E-mail address: zinsj@ccf.org

Clin Plastic Surg 49 (2022) 339–348
https://doi.org/10.1016/j.cps.2022.03.001

position exist that help to guide our surgical decision-making when analyzing the brow for rejuvenation.

The modern description of brow position was described by Westmore in 1974.[1] The medial brow originates on the same vertical plane as the lateral alar border and medial canthus. Here, it is rounded in shape and has the greatest density of hair follicles. In females, the brow continues laterally to form a gentle arch that peaks at the junction between its lateral and middle third, aligning at the lateral limbus. The space between the upper eyelid crease and the brow should gradually increase from medial to lateral.[2] Debate exists in the literature regarding ideal vertical brow position in females, but at least 5 mm above the rim is the esthetic ideal.[3-5] From medial to lateral, brow thickness decreases to a taper at the tail of the brow, which is positioned along an oblique line connecting the ipsilateral nasal ala and lateral canthus. In females, the tail of the brow should sit in a slightly higher vertical position than the medial origin.[6] The male brow tends to be flatter with less of an arch, traveling at the level of the superior orbital rim. Although it still tapers laterally, hair density tends to be more uniform and fuller throughout its length. It is suggested that the term brow lifting is inaccurate and a misnomer. A better description of brow rejuvenation would be "shaping" (**Fig. 1**).

BROW AGING

The brow's contribution to periorbital aging is often times underappreciated. Although upper eyelid dermatochalasis, development of crow's feet, and glabellar rhytids are important areas for treatment, they rarely occur in isolation. Brow ptosis is defined by a loss of vertical position of the brow relative to the supraorbital rim, giving a heavy and tired appearance to the eyes. Observational studies by Lambros have shown that the brow position descends with age.[7] In addition, the shape of the brow also undergoes significant change. The gentle arch and peak are lost as the brow becomes flatter.[8] Importantly, the medial brow is more fixed and less mobile than the lateral brow. Therefore, descent of the lateral brow below the level of the medial brow is a common feature of aging. Work by Matros and colleagues[9] demonstrated this phenomenon by showing little change in medial brow position between youthful and aged patient cohorts. Cadaver studies by Knize illustrate the anatomic basis for higher susceptibility of the lateral brow to descend with age.[10] Specifically, greater mobility of the lateral brow is afforded by the galeal fat pad, the

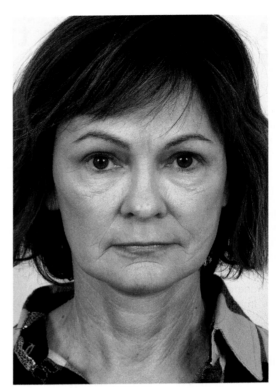

Fig. 1. The medial brow originates on the same vertical plane as the lateral alar base. In the female, it forms a gentle superior arc from medial to lateral with the apex of the arc at the lateral limbus or junction of the middle and lateral third of the brow. In the male, the ideal brow shape is flatter, lower, and located at the superior orbital rim.

preseptal fat pad, and the subgaleal glide plane. The lack of the presence of the frontalis muscle laterally allows the lateral orbicularis oculi to act relatively unimpeded. The medial brow on the other hand remains more fixed and less mobile with strong glabellar muscle attachment with no significant associated fat pads or gliding plane. As a result, the lateral brow descends with age, often resulting in compensatory frontalis hyperactivity (**Fig. 2**).

Correction of this lateral descent is a primary goal of surgical and nonsurgical treatment and also effects the longevity of surgical intervention. Relapse following surgical correction most commonly occurs at the tail of the brow owing to the depressor action of the lateral orbicularis oculi and the absence of frontalis antagonistic effect.[11] Medial brow ptosis may also be addressed in some patients, but rarely is medial correction alone indicated. With descent, lateral hooding occurs and is commonly mistaken for excess upper eyelid skin. Performing a blepharoplasty alone in

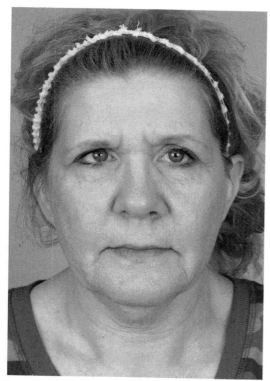

Fig. 2. Brow aging and loss of brow shape. The lateral brow descends to a greater degree than the medial brow. When the lateral brow is lower than the medial brow, the patient has a sad or tired appearance.

these patients cannot correct lateral brow hooding. Bruneau and colleagues[12] have shown that with aging, a lower brow position is associated with the presence of dermatochalasis, as well as compensatory frontalis hyperactivity. In some cases, brow ptosis may be severe enough to cause a superior lateral visual field loss. In such cases, ptosis visual field testing to document and confirm a field deficit may lead to insurance coverage. Finally, the heavy brow may lead to pseudoptosis which may be corrected by brow surgery alone. In addition, unrecognized upper eyelid ptosis may accompany brow ptosis and, if so, requires correction. Accurately distinguishing between upper eyelid ptosis, upper eyelid dermatochalasis, and brow ptosis is critical as is recognizing their concomitant occurrence.

THE FOREHEAD

The forehead comprises the upper third of an esthetically balanced face and includes the eyebrows. Its well-defined layers have an important impact on the various surgical planes of dissection. They include the skin, subcutaneous tissue, galeal frontalis muscle, loose areolar tissue plane that is relatively avascular, and periosteum. The galea in particularly has been well described by Knize.[13] It is composed of a superficial and deep portion that encases the frontalis muscle beginning at its origin. More inferiorly, the deep galea splits into a superficial and deep layer enveloping the galeal fat pad which continues below the level of the brow. In the lowest portion of the forehead, the deep galea splits once again, forming a gliding plane coinciding with the transverse portion of the corrugator muscle. This gliding plane affords the brow its high degree of dynamic motion during expression. The deepest layer then fuses with periosteum just above the supraorbital rim (**Fig. 3**).

Anatomy of the temporal area is similarly complex but mirrors the anatomy of the forehead just described. Understanding this three-dimensional anatomy is critical to avoid injury to the frontal branch of the facial nerve. In the temple the superficial temporal fascia, or temporoparietal fascia, lies immediately superficial to the skin and subcutaneous tissue. Deep to the superficial temporal fascia lies the deep temporal fascia which is a single layer covering the temporalis muscle. Proceeding inferiorly, approximately at the level of the brow, the deep temporal fascia splits to form the superficial and deep layers of the deep temporal fascia. This can be recognized because of a color change. Superiorly the deep temporal fascia is red in color, reflecting the temporalis muscle. Inferiorly the superficial and deep layers of the deep temporal fascia invest the intermediate fat pad. This gives this area its characteristic yellow color[14] (**Fig. 4**).

In women, 6-7 cm is the esthetic ideal for vertical forehead length measured from the trichion to the glabella. Deviation from these proportions may classify the forehead as either long or short and convex or flat. Brow shape and height play a decisive role in choosing the most appropriate technique for brow lift surgery.[15] Rhytids are oriented transversely, lying perpendicular to the frontalis muscle fibers. Variability in the hairline may exist. A midline peak or "widow's peak" is congenital and should be noted when present. With age, irregularities in the hairline tend to develop, with temporal recession common in most males but not infrequent in middle-aged females. In addition to the changes in hairline, an aged forehead may be marked by deep, resting rhytids and diffuse actinic changes through accumulated sun exposure.[16] In men, the forehead is higher than in women, especially with recession of the anterior hairline. Males are classified as having "stronger" foreheads, attributable primarily to bossing at the frontal sinus, giving the appearance of a heavy brow ridge. The superior lateral orbital rim tends to be more prominent than in the female.

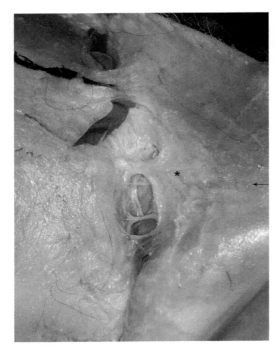

Fig. 3. The frontalis muscle is invested on its deep and superficial surface by the superficial and deep layers of the galea. Inferiorly the deep layer splits to invest the galeal fat pad on its superficial and deep surfaces. In the lowest portion, the deep galea splits once more forming the gliding plane with the corrugator muscle. Finally the deep layer fuses with the periosteum just above the orbital rim.

Transverse rhytids are also characteristically deeper and more pronounced, while the general nature of the skin tends to be more sebaceous[17] (**Fig. 5**).

BONY ANATOMY AND ZONES OF FIXATION

The frontal bone composes most of the forehead, with the supraorbital rim acting as a constant bony landmark to assess brow position and ptosis. At the lateral margin of the frontal bone lies the superior temple fusion line or temporal crest. This marks the transition point from the forehead medially to the temporal fossa laterally. The superior temporal line can be identified by having the patient bight down. The line of fusion is just superior to the contracting temporalis muscle (**Fig. 6**). The line of fusion is approximately 5 mm in width throughout the length of the ridge.[13] It includes a confluence of the galea aponeurotica and its lateral continuation the superficial temporal fascia, as well as the deep temporal fascia. Immediately medial to this line of fusion, it is important to dissect in the subperiosteal plane to avoid injury to the deep branch of the supraorbital nerve (**Fig. 7**). Approaching the orbital rim, the zone of adhesion becomes denser and expands to form the temporal ligamentous adhesion or orbital ligament. This dense fascial convergence connects the superficial temporal fascia to the orbital rim at the tail of the brow and is continuous with the lateral orbital thickening at the lateral orbital rim. Surgical release of these areas where soft tissue is adherent to bone represents a key principle in

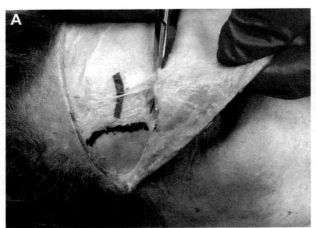

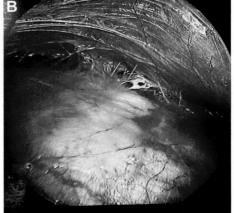

Fig. 4. (*A*) Cadaver dissection demonstrating the deep temporal fascia (red) covering the temporalis muscle (*arrow*). Inferiorly the color changes to yellow as the deep temporal fascia splits to form the superficial and deep layers of the deep temporal fascia investing the intermediate fat pad (*asterisk*). (*B*) Endoscopic view of the same structures. Superiorly (three o'clock) the deep temporal fascia appears red, reflecting the underlying temporalis muscle. Inferiorly the yellow color indicates that the deep temporal fascia has split into the superficial and deep layers of the deep temporal fascia, investing the yellow intermediate fat pad.

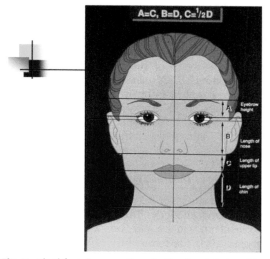

Fig. 5. Ideal facial proportions in the frontal view. The face can be divided into thirds. Distance A (brow to medial canthus) is roughly equal to the vertical distance of the upper lip (C). Distance B (midface) is roughly equal to the distance from the alar base to the inferior border of the chin (D).

effective brow lift surgery (see **Fig. 7**). As mentioned previously, the medial eyebrow is significantly less mobile than the lateral brow, attributable to the more robust muscle attachments comprising the galea and anchoring from the supraorbital and supratrochlear neurovascular bundles.[10]

MUSCLES

Brow animation plays a distinctive role in the display of emotion. Medial depression with furrowing signals anger or disagreement, exaggerated elevation suggests surprise and excitement, and lateral depression is associated with sadness. Unilateral elevation is synonymous with skeptical curiosity or intrigue in today's popular culture. Maintaining an ability to animate the brow after surgery avoids the frozen and perpetually surprised appearance that is often negatively associated with an overoperated result.[18]

The muscles of facial expression that are responsible for brow movement represent dynamic and opposing forces. A variety of brow depressors act across the lower forehead, whereas the frontalis muscle stands as the sole brow elevator. Manipulation of these forces through neuromodulation or surgical muscle excision can generate desirable changes in brow position.

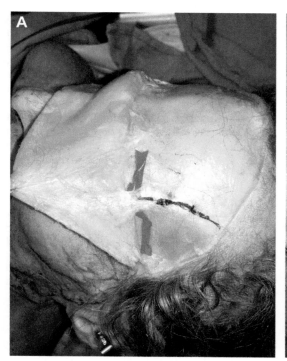

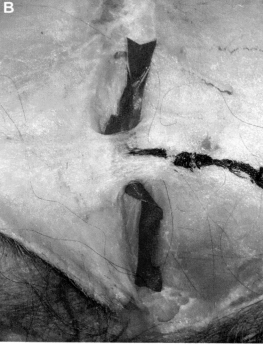

Fig. 6. (*A*) Cadaver dissection demonstrating the superior temporal fusion line marked in blue. If the fusion line is followed caudally, it coalesces with the temporal ligamentous adhesion. This fascial fusion must be divided to elevate the lateral brow. (*B*) Close up of (*A*) demonstrating the temporal ligamentous adhesion.

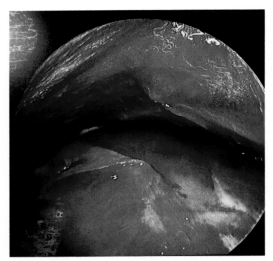

Fig. 7. Endoscopic view of the right temporal fusion line identified and dissection then medially immediately taken subperiosteal to avoid injury to the deep branch of the supraorbital nerve.

Specifically weakening of the depressor muscles can allow the frontalis to act relatively unopposed leading to brow elevation. Conversely, weakening of the frontalis especially in the lower forehead can inadvertently lead to eyebrow ptosis. Strong muscle action produces distinct and predictable rhytides perpendicular to the muscle fibers which are accentuated with age. It is important to distinguish rhytides as either dynamic or static to determine the most effective treatment modality. Static rhytides will not respond well to neuromodulation, whereas dynamic rhytides will.

Brow Elevation

The frontalis muscle is a broad, thin muscle fanning across the forehead and terminating at the superior temporal septum. Originating at the galea superiorly at the approximate level of the hairline, it inserts into the dermis at the eyebrow. Inferiorly, it interdigitates with the opposing procerus and orbicularis oculi muscles. Laterally, it fuses at the temporal crests.[13] Therefore, because it is absent laterally, it provides no counteraction to the depressor activity of the lateral orbicularis. When activated, the frontalis is responsible for transverse forehead rhytids. Identifying the location of these forehead wrinkles also gives insight into the decussation pattern of the muscle in the midline. According to anatomic cadaver studies by Raveendran, it was most common for some degree of decussation to exist. However, approximately 1 in 4 specimens demonstrate complete separation between the two muscle bellies.

When present, decussation either occurred at the level of the brow or continued to the mid forehead. They suggest that variability may exist based on ethnicity and contribute to the general shape differences of the periorbital region between cultures.[19] Of clinical importance, identifying the extent of frontalis muscle proper in the midline helps to guide treatment with neuromodulators to avoid residual dynamic rhytids, asymmetry, and iatrogenic brow ptosis following injection.[20]

Medial Brow Depression: The Glabella

A series of muscles act to pull the medial brow medially and inferiorly. They originate from bone and insert at various locations into dermis. Their action causes the formation of distinct rhytids at the glabella which are a hallmark of facial aging.[10] The procerus muscle forms at the superior aspect of the nasal bones and runs vertically, producing transverse rhytids at the bridge of the nose. The corrugator supercilia begins at the superomedial orbital rim and travels primarily in a transverse orientation, forming the vertical or "eleven lines" at the glabella. Anatomically, evidence of a transverse and oblique head of the corrugator supercilia have been described but are many times indistinct from one another clinically[21,22] (**Fig. 8**). The orbicularis oculi muscle is arranged as a sphincter surrounding the orbit. Originating at the medial canthal tendon, the superomedial orbital portion is arranged obliquely, pulling the brow inferomedially. This assists with voluntary eyelid closure. In addition, the depressor supercilii muscle has been described in cadaver studies as a distinct medial brow depressor from the corrugator supercilii and orbicularis muscle, oriented obliquely but more vertically relative to the orbicularis. Its origin is relatively low, at the frontal process of the maxilla approximately 1 cm above the medial canthal tendon. At this origin, the angular artery passes within its fibers.[23]

Lateral Brow Depression

The lateral portion of the orbicularis oculi is solely responsible for lateral brow depression. As it inserts at the lateral orbital thickening, its fibers are primarily vertical, forming the rhytids associated with "crow's feet"[10] (**Fig. 9**).

NEUROVASCULAR STRUCTURES

The muscles of facial expression responsible for brow movement receive innervation from specific branches of the facial nerve. The frontal branch powers the frontalis muscle to elevate the brow

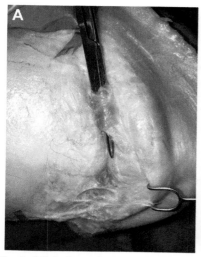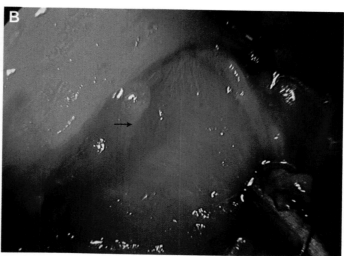

Fig. 8. (A) Cadaver dissection of the corrugator muscle. The muscle is best approached subgaleally or subperiosteally. Anatomically it has a transverse and oblique head. Within the muscle lie the suprtrochlear nerve branches. (B) Endoscopic view of the left corrugator muscle partially excised in the center of the photograph. Distal cut end of the muscle is marked with an arrow. Endoscopic grasper is visualized in the lower right.

and have been studied extensively. Pitanguy and Ramos originally described the trajectory of the frontal branch of the facial nerve along a line projected from a point 0.5 cm below the tragus to a point 1.5 cm above the tail of the brow.[24] At the zygomatic arch, this correlates to the middle third of the arch, approximately 4 cm from the lateral canthus. The frontal branch remains in a plane deep to the parotidmasseteric fascia until crossing the arch. Cadaver dissections by Agarwal and colleagues[25] identify a fascial transition zone 1.5 to 3.0 cm above the arch and 0.9 to 1.4 cm posterior to the lateral orbital rim where the frontal branch then passes from the innominate fascia to run within the superficial temporal fascia. For this reason, staying deep or immediately on top of the superficial layer of the deep temporal fascia avoids injury to this nerve branch within the temporal fossa. It should be noted that some terminal branches of the frontal nerve do play a role in innervating medial brow depressors, primarily the transverse portion of the corrugator supercilii and procerus. However, these contributions are both minor and redundant. If an injury to the frontal branch is sustained, iatrogenic brow ptosis and asymmetry result.[26] While a variety of muscles act synergistically to depress the brow, all share primary innervation by the zygomatic branch of the facial nerve on their deep surface. Although the buccal branch plays an important functional component in innervating the palpebral portion of the orbicularis oculi muscle, this action has no effect on brow position.[27] Alghoul and colleagues

have shown that the upper zygomatic branch of the facial nerve to be found consistently deep to the upper third of the zygomatic major muscle in the sub-superficial musculo aponeurotic system (SMAS) plane. It continues medially to innervate the medial brow depressors of the glabella.[28]

Sensory innervation to the forehead and brow relies on the supraorbital and supratrochlear nerves, both branches from the ophthalmic division of the trigeminal nerve. The supratrochlear

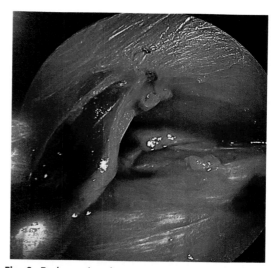

Fig. 9. Endoscopic subperiosteal dissection along the lateral orbital rim releases all soft tissue of the rim except for the deep head of the lateral canthal tendon.

neurovascular bundle may be found approximately 1.5 cm on average from midline as it emerges from a bony notch or foramen at the supraorbital rim.[29] It runs through the medial aspect of the corrugator muscle dividing into multiple branches as it provides sensation to the inferior medial forehead and glabella. Clinically, nerve branches are skeletonized during corrugator resection[30] (see **Fig. 8**B). The supraorbital nerve is found lateral to the supratrochlear nerve, originating approximately 2.5 cm from the midline as it emerges from the supraorbital notch or foramen[31] (**Fig. 10**). Often times, this is a distinct, palpable bony landmark. In 90% of cases, a true notch exists although a true bony foramen located up to 1.5 cm cephalad to the supraorbital rim may be present 10% of the time. The supraorbital nerve then divides immediately into a deep and superficial branch. The superficial division travels superior medially, passing through the frontalis muscle into the subcutaneous plane in the mid to upper central forehead. The deep division runs superior laterally, staying deep to the galea on top of periosteum. Within 0.5 to 1.5 cm medial, it then remains parallel to the temporal crest (**Fig. 11**). Along this course, branches emerge that pierce the galea sequentially, providing sensation to the frontoparietal scalp.[32] Because the nerve lies between galea and periosteum, it is readily injured during a subgaleal dissection. This can lead to chronic and intractable pruritus of the scalp.

Vascular supply to the brow and forehead is robust and derived from both the internal and external carotid systems. Centrally, the

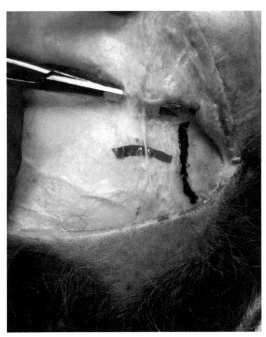

Fig. 11. Cadaver dissection demonstrating the deep branch of the supraorbital nerve coursing 0.5 to 1.5 cm medial to the superior temporal fusion line. The deep branch lies between periosteum and galea and is easily injured in a subgaleal dissection.

supraorbital and supratrochlear neurovascular bundles form from the ophthalmic artery of the internal carotid. Laterally, the superficial temporal artery represents the terminal branch of the

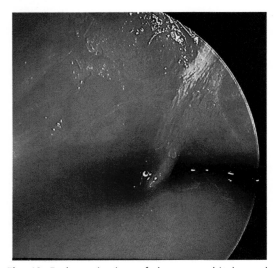

Fig. 10. Endoscopic view of the supraorbital vessels emanating from the supraorbital foramen 2.5 cm from the midline.

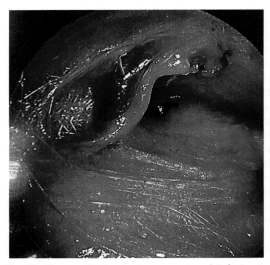

Fig. 12. The sentinel vein is encountered inferior to the inferior temporal septum. It lies 1.5 cm lateral and 2 cm superior to the lateral orbital rim. The frontal branch of the facial nerve is superior and lateral to the vein.

external carotid, transmitting frontal branches to the forehead. Of note, the sentinel vein is an important vascular landmark during surgical brow lifting. Cadaver studies have demonstrated its consistent location, superior lateral to the lateral orbital rim passing from the subcutaneous layer through the superficial temporal fascia and then deep temporal fascia into the temporalis muscle.[33–35] Work by Yang and colleagues[36] show a reliable superficial origin by marking a point 1.5 cm lateral and 2 cm superior to the lateral orbital rim. This vessel consistently lies inferior and anterior to the frontal branch of the facial nerve. Therefore, once the sentinel vein is encountered, the lateral dissection of the brow has passed the frontal branch of the facial nerve[34] **(Fig. 12)**.

SUMMARY

The brow is a dynamic structure with distinct youthful features. With age, predictable changes occur to its position and shape. In mastering the various means of correcting the aging brow, a

---

- Loss of the natural shape of the superior lateral orbit occurs with aging. Elevation of the lateral brow is the best means of correction
- Lateral brow elevation requires release of the superior temporal septum and temporal ligamentous adhesion
- Injury to the deep branch of the supraorbital nerve is common in the subgaleal approach and is avoided by understanding of the pertinent anatomy. Subperiosteal dissection in this region minimizes the risk
- Frontal branch injury during temporal dissection is prevented by staying deep to or directly on top of the superficial layer of the deep temporal fascia in the temporal region.
- In resecting the corrugator muscle, the branches of the supratrochlear nerve will be encountered and should be preserved.

---

thorough understanding of the complex anatomy of the periorbita, forehead, and temple is essential if superior results are to be obtained and complications minimized.

CLINICS CARE POINTS

DISCLOSURE

The authors have nothing to disclose.

REFERENCES

1. Westmore MG. Facial cosmetics in conjunction with surgery. Course presented at the aesthetic plastic surgery society meeting. Vancouver: British Columbia; 1975.
2. Alghoul MS, Bricker JT, Venkatesh V, et al. Rethinking upper blepharoplasty: the impact of pretarsal show. Plast Reconstr Surg 2020;146(6): 1239–47.
3. Matarasso A, Terino EO. Forehead-brow rhytidoplasty: reassessing the goals. Plast Reconstr Surg 1994;93(7):1378–91.
4. McKinney P, Mossie RD, Zukowski ML. Criteria for the forehead lift. Aesthetic Plast Surg 1991;15(2): 141–7.
5. Gunter JP, Antrobus SD. Aesthetic analysis of the eyebrows. Plast Reconstr Surg 1997;99:1807.
6. Fruend RM, Nolan WB. Correlation between brow lift outcomes and aesthetic ideals for eyebrow height and shape in females. Plast Reconstr Surg 1996; 97:1343.
7. Lambros V. Observations on periorbital and midface aging. Plast Reconstr Surg 2007;120(5):1367–76.
8. Codner MA, Kikkawa DO, Korn BS, et al. Blepharoplasty and brow lift. Plast Reconstr Surg 2010;126: 1e.
9. Matros E, Garcia JA, Yaremchuk MJ. Changes in eyebrow position and shape with aging. Plast Reconstr Surg 2009;124(4):1296–301.
10. Knize DM. An anatomically based study of the mechanism of eyebrow ptosis. Plast Reconstr Surg 1996;97:1321.
11. Jones BM, Lo SJ. The impact of endoscopic brow lift on eyebrow morphology, aesthetics, and longevity. Plast Reconstr Surg 2013;132(2):226e–38e.
12. Bruneau SM, Foletti JM, Muller S, et al. Does the eyebrow sag with aging? An anthopometric study of 95 caucasians from 20 to 79 years of age. Plast Reconstr Surg 2016;132(2):305e–12e.
13. Knize DM, editor. The forehead and temporal fossa: anatomy and technique. Philadelphia: Lippincott Williams & Wilkins; 2001.
14. Stuzin JM, Wagstrom L, Kawamoto HK, et al. Anatomy of the frontal branch of the facial nerve: the significance of the temporal fat pad. Plast Reconstr Surg 1989;83(2):265–71.
15. Guyuron B, Lee M. A reappraisal of surgical techniques and efficacy in forehead rejuvenation. Plast Reconstr Surg 2014;134(3):426–35.
16. Knoll BI, Attkiss KJ, Persing JA. The influence of forehead, brow, and periorbital aesthetics on perceived expression in the youthful face. Plast Reconstr Surg 2008;121(5):1793–802.
17. Knize DM. Anatomic concepts for brow lift procedures. Plast Reconstr Surg 2009;124:2118.

18. Yaremchuk MJ, O'Sullivan N, Benslimane F. Reversing brow lifts. Aesthet Surg J 2007;27(4): 367–75.

19. Raveendran SS, Anthony DJ. Classification and morphological variation of the frontalis muscle and implications on the clinical practice. Aesthet Plast Surg 2021;45(1):164–70.

20. Jabbour SF, Awaida CJ, ElKhoury JS, et al. The impact of upper face botulinum toxin injections on eyebrow height and forehead lines: a randomized controlled trial and an algorithmic approach to forehead injection. Plast Reconstr Surg 2018;142(5): 1212–7.

21. Janis JE, Ghavami A, Lemmon JA, et al. Anatomy of the corrugator supercilii muscle: part I. Corrugator topography. Plast Reconstr Surg 2007;120:1647.

22. Knize DM. Muscles that act on glabellar skin: a closer look. Plast Reconstr Surg 2000;105(1): 350–61.

23. Cook BE Jr, Lucarelli MJ, Lemke BN. Depressor supercilii muscle: anatomy, histology, and cosmetic implications. Ophthalmic Plast Reconstr Surg 2001; 17(6):404–11.

24. Pitanguy I, Ramos S. The frontal branch of the facial nerve: the importance of its variations in facelifting. Plast Reconstr Surg 1966;38:352–6.

25. Agarwal CA, Mendenhall SD 3rd, Foreman KB, et al. The course of the frontal branch of the facial nerve in relation to fascial planes: an anatomic study. Plast Reconstr Surg 2010;125(2):532–7.

26. Roostaeian J, Rohrich RJ, Stuzin JM. Anatomical considerations to prevent facial nerve injury. Plast Reconstr Surg 2015;135(5):1318–27.

27. Hwang K. Facial nerve supply to the orbicularis oculi around the lower eyelid: anatomy and its clinical implications. Plast Reconstr Surg 2018;141(3): 449e–50e.

28. Alghoul M, Bitik O, McBride J, et al. Relationship of the zygomaticofacial nerve to the retaining ligaments of the face: the Sub-SMAS Danger Zone. Plast Reconstr Surg 2013;131(2):245e-52e.

29. Miller TM, Rudkin G, Honig M, et al. Lateral subcutaneous brow lift and interbrow muscle resection: clinical experience and anatomic studies. Plast Reconstr Surg 2000;105:1120–7.

30. Janis JE, Hatef DA, Hagan R, et al. Anatomy of the supratrochlear nerve: implications for the surgical treatment of migraine headaches. Plast Reconstr Surg 2013;131:743.

31. Knize DM. A study of the supraorbital nerve. Plast Reconstr Surg 1995;96:564.

32. Janis JE, Ghavami A, Lemmon JA, et al. The anatomy of the corrugator supercilii muscle: part II. Supraorbital nerve branching patterns. Plast Reconstr Surg 2008;121:233.

33. Plaza R, Valiente E, Arroyo JM. Supraperiosteal lifting of the upper two-thirds of the face. Br J Plast Surg 1991;44:325–32.

34. Trinei FA, Januszkiewicz J, Nahai F. The sentinel vein: an important reference point for surgery in the temporal region. Plast Reconstr Surg 1998; 101(1):27–32.

35. Friedman T, Lurie D, Westreich M. Rembrandt's sentinel vein. Aesth Surg J 2007;27(1):105–7.

36. Yang H, Jung W, Won S, et al. Anatomical study of medial zygomaticotemporal vein and its clinical implication regarding the injectable treatments. Surg Radiol Anat 2014;37:175–80.

The Hairline Brow Lift

James Walter Dutton Jr, MD[a], Irene A. Chang, BA[b], James E. Zins, MD, FACS[a,c],*

KEY WORDS

• Hairline brow lift • Pretrichial incision • Brow lift • Brow ptosis • Facial rejuvenation

KEY POINTS

- Description of brow lift indications and contraindications.
- Comparisons of hairline brow lift with other open and endoscopic techniques.
- Detailed description of surgical technique.
- Description of modifications of technique.

 Video content accompanies this article at http://www.plasticsurgery.theclinics.com.

INTRODUCTION

Brow ptosis is an early manifestation of an aging forehead and can contribute to patients appearing tired or angry. Effective rejuvenation of the upper face results when effective brow repositioning is combined with maintenance or improvement of brow shape.

Classically brow ptosis was treated with an open coronal brow lift. However, this technique has generally fallen out of favor for several reasons. It may elevate the hairline and vertically lengthen the upper face. However, its greatest drawback is the substantial hairline incision, and the potential for scalp hypesthesia, pruritis, and alopecia.[1,2] Pretrichial or hairline brow lifts allow surgeons to address all aspects of forehead and brow aging and is performed in subperiosteal, subgaleal, or subcutaneous planes. Hairline brow lifts avoid vertical forehead lengthening and allow for forehead reduction in patients with high hairlines while simultaneously allowing more precise brow elevation when compared with the coronal approach.[3]

Other open techniques, such as direct and temporal lifts, have also been used to improve brow position. Direct brow lifts allow for precise brow elevation through excision of full thickness skin directly above the brow while preserving scalp and forehead sensation. Although direct brow lifts have traditionally been reserved for older men with deep forehead crease and high hairlines, Pelle-Ceravolo and Angelini[4] have demonstrated excellent results with this technique in a large and diverse patient cohort. Temporal brow lifts also use skin excision to elevate the lateral brow. Temporal brow lifts are advantageous because of immediate scar camouflage provided by temporal hair and can significantly improve lateral brow hooding.[5] However, unlike the pretrichial approach, temporal brow lifts address lateral brow ptosis and do not address corrugator hyperactivity. Therefore if the corrugators are to be addressed additional techniques must be added. Furthermore, direct and temporal brow lifts only address lateral brow ptosis and do not improve medial brow position or address horizontal forehead rhytids in the midforehead.

Endoscopic brow lift techniques have increased in popularity as surgeons have investigated less invasive surgical procedures. Endoscopic techniques are performed through a series of three to five small incisions well hidden in the hair avoiding the significant coronal incision while addressing most aspects of forehead and brow aging. Endoscopic techniques also avoid vertical forehead

[a] Cleveland Clinic Department of Plastic Surgery, 9500 Euclid Avenue, Cleveland, OH 44195-0001, USA; [b] Case Western Reserve School of Medicine Health Education Campus, 9501 Eucllid Avenue, Cleveland, OH 44106, USA; [c] Section of Cosmetic Surgery, Cleveland Clinic Plastic Surgery, 9500 Euclid Avenue, Cleveland, OH 44195-0001, USA
* Corresponding author. Cleveland Clinic Department of Plastic Surgery, 9500 Euclid Avenue, Cleveland, OH 44195-0001.
E-mail address: Zinsj@ccf.org

Clin Plastic Surg 49 (2022) 349–356
https://doi.org/10.1016/j.cps.2022.01.004

lengthening while preserving the hairline and forehead sensation. The principal disadvantages of endoscopic lifts include increased technical demand with the use of endoscopic equipment, inability to fine tune brow position, and questionable longevity of resultant brow position compared with the hairline brow approach.[4,6] The ideal candidates for the endoscopic lift are thus patients with a short or normal forehead length, a straight forehead, and no true medial skin excess. Less ideal candidates are those with a high or convex forehead, thinning hairline, deep forehead wrinkles, or true medial skin excess.

PATIENT SELECTION

Patient assessment should be done with the patient sitting or standing with the head in a vertical position. Similarly to all brow lift operations, surgeons must assess the patient for eyebrow symmetry, shape, position of the anterior hairline, scalp hair thickness, temporal hooding, corrugator and procerus activity, and the presence of true medial skin excess.

INDICATIONS

One of the most important determinants in the decision to use a pretrichial incision is the presence of medial and lateral brow ptosis. The hairline incision allows surgeons to address global brow ptosis unlike endoscopic or more limited open incision techniques, such as the temporal brow lift, which only address lateral brow ptosis.[7] An example of a patient with medial and lateral brow ptosis preoperatively and the result after hairline brow lift is seen in **Figs. 1–3**.

Ideal candidates are those patients with high frontal hairlines who would benefit from hairline lowering. The high forehead is defined at 7 cm or greater from the lateral third of the eyebrow to the anterior hairline. When using the pretrichial incision in those patients for whom hairline lowering is planned, the posterior dissection is performed in the subgaleal plane to minimize the likelihood of hair loss. Bony fixation is often used to maintain the new hairline position.[8–10] Alternatively, hairline brow lifts may be used in patients with overly high eyebrows, which may be a result of congenital or previous brow lift surgeries. In patients where the hairline approach is used to lower the eyebrow position, bony fixation is performed at multiple levels to minimize late loss of scalp advancement.[11]

The hairline brow lift is also effective in addressing deep forehead rhytids in patients desiring forehead rejuvenation. Dissection is carried out through the subcutaneous plane, which allows for release of fibrous dermal attachments that may be contributing to transverse forehead wrinkles, as seen in **Fig. 4**. The dissection is performed in the subcutaneous plane to the most caudal horizontal forehead wrinkle is released, and then the dissection may transition planes to deep to frontalis medially to expose corrugator and procerus muscles allowing exposure and resection of glabellar musculature to address rhytids in this region. In this setting, the subcutaneous dissection is continued laterally to the lateral eyebrow.[12] Deep vertical rhytids in the glabellar region may be further treated with superficial autologous fat injections to aid in rejuvenation of this area.[13,14]

CONTRAINDICATIONS

One of the primary contraindications of pretrichial incisions are patients who find the anterior hairline incision unacceptable and desire entirely concealable postoperative scarring. Such techniques as placing the incision a few millimeters posterior to hairline, acute beveling of incision, and cutting across hairline follicles to maximize hair grow along scar can improve the appearance of the anterior hairline scar. This approach can create a cosmetically acceptable postoperative scar appearance. However, a thorough discussion of scar placement and outcomes should occur before performing this technique in any patient.[15] Hairline scars of consecutive anterior hairline brow lift patients are demonstrated in **Figs. 5–7**.

Pretrichial incisions should also be avoided in patients with short forehead distances because this procedure further shortens the distance between the hairline and eyebrow position. Patients with short forehead distances of low hairlines who may require hairline elevation are better served with brow lift techniques that either maintain forehead distance, such as endoscopic brow lift, or even elevate the hairline, such as coronal brow lift.

TECHNIQUE

The hairline brow lift is performed under local anesthesia, intravenous sedation, or general anesthetic.

The pretrichial incision is designed 2 to 5 mm within the hairline for best means of camouflage. The incision extends across the frontal hairline until it reaches the hairline laterally as it transitions into hair-bearing temporal scalp. Unless hairline lowering is planned the incision does not extend beyond the level of the superior temporal line or crest. Scar visibility is minimized by using a

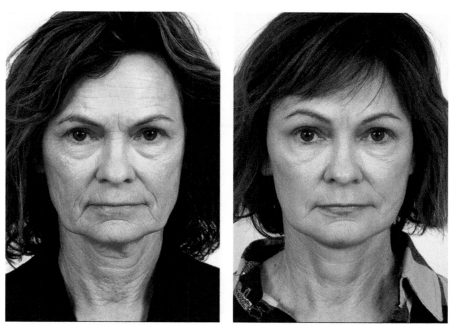

Fig. 1. Patient with preoperative medial and lateral brow ptosis (*left*) and postoperative results (*right*) 3 months after facelift, neck lift, perioral chemical peel, and full hairline brow lift with global brow elevation.

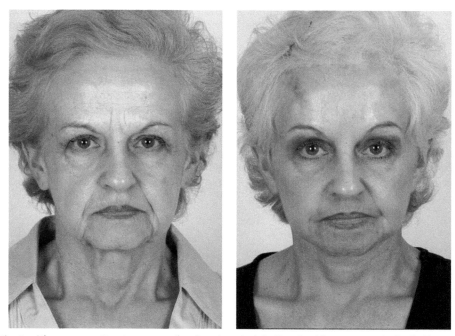

Fig. 2. Patient with preoperative transverse forehead and glabellar rhytids preoperatively (*left*). Postoperative appearance (*right*) 6 months after hairline brow lift, extended superficial musculoaponeurotic system facelift, and perioral croton oil peel showing uniform improvement in rhytids and improved brow contour and position 6 months after hairline brow lift, extended superficial musculoaponeurotic system facelift, and perioral croton oil peel.

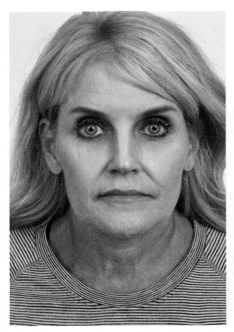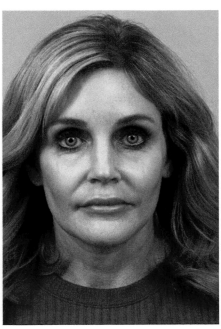

Fig. 3. Patient with preoperative medial and lateral brow ptosis (*left*) and postoperative results (*right*) 2 months after facelift, neck lift, perioral croton oil peel, and full hairline brow lift with improved brow position and contour.

wavy, random pattern or alternatively in a zigzag fashion according to surgeon preference.

A beveled incision is used to promote hair growth through the resultant scar. Although the dissection is carried out in the subcutaneous, subgaleal, or subperiosteal plane, the subcutaneous route is ideal because this is where elevation of the brow is most readily accomplished. Regardless of plane, the dissection is carried down until the brow is mobilized from its supraorbital attachments medially and laterally taking care to preserve supraorbital and supratrochlear nerves and vasculature.

After mobilization of the forehead and brow, the forehead skin is advanced and the redundant forehead skin is measured and excised. In patients with particularly long foreheads, further forehead reduction and lowering of the hairline is achieved through concurrent subgaleal dissection posteriorly toward the vertex of the skull allowing mobilization of the scalp. The posterior scalp flap advancement is augmented by galeal scoring, which includes transverse incisions through the galea taking care to preserve subcutaneous scalp vasculature. This allows for more dramatic anterior advancement of the frontal scalp before closure.

After adequate hemostasis, the incision is then closed in layers with either a deep dermal or galeal suture in combination with a skin suture for precise realignment.

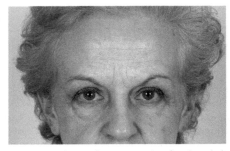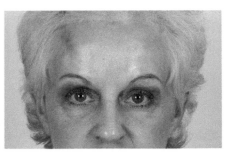

Fig. 4. Patient comparison of preoperative forehead rhytids (*left*) and postoperative result (*left*) 6 months after hairline brow lift showing improved transverse forehead rhytids and brow position and contour.

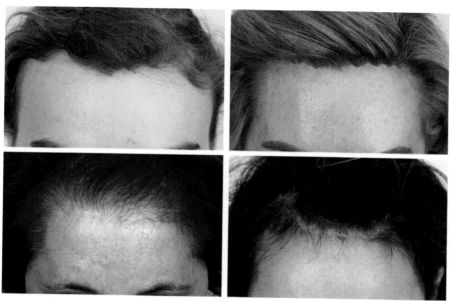

Fig. 5. Four consecutive patient examples who had hairline brow lift performed and resultant scar appearance.

AUTHORS' PREFERRED TECHNIQUE

A zigzag incision is designed a few millimeters posterior to the anterior hairline extending from the temporal hair bearing scalp bilaterally. Before incision, the incision and forehead are tumesced using 0.5% lidocaine with 1:200,000 epinephrine mixed with 2 mg of tranexamic acid per cubic centimeter of local anesthetic to minimize bleeding and improve visualization. Tranexamic acid comes in a 10-mL vial of 100 mg/cc. Therefore to obtain this dilution 2 mL of 100 mg/cc of tranexamic acid is mixed with 100 mL of 0.5% lidocaine. We have found tranexamic acid mixed with local anesthesia and injected in this fashion produces profoundly dry surgical field and results in minimal postoperative bruising.[16]

After allowing adequate time for epinephrine effect, a scalpel is used to create an exaggerated bevel incision to preserve hair follicles [Video 1].

The incision is carried down until the superficial portion of the frontalis muscle is visualized. Under direct visualization a combination of blunt and sharp dissection is used to elevate the forehead in a subcutaneous plane just above the frontalis muscle [**Fig 8**, Video 2]. A blunt or blind dissection in the subcutaneous plane has been previously described, but in the authors' experience these techniques often result in violation of the frontalis muscle and increased possibility for bleeding.[17] The dissection is carried inferiorly until the medial and lateral brow are completely elevated from their supraorbital periosteal attachments and the brow is fully mobilized [Video 3]. The resultant forehead flap is then positioned posteriorly and the redundant forehead skin is then measured and excised in an identical zigzag pattern to the initial incision using Zins clamp [Video 3].[18] After meticulous hemostasis, the incision is then closed in layers with 3–0 Monocryl deep dermal sutures followed by 5–

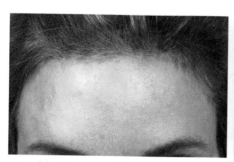
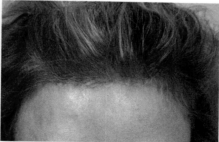

Fig. 6. Closeup of hairline brow lift scar appearance 2 months postoperative.

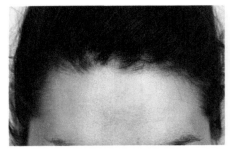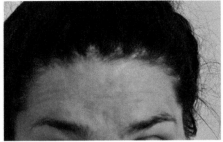

Fig. 7. Closeup of gender reassignment male to female patient preoperatively (*left*) and postoperative result (*right*) 2 years status post hairline brow lift with resultant scar appearance.

0 Prolene sutures placed as half-buried horizontal mattress sutures with the transcutaneous portion of the mattress placed on the scalp side to minimize scar inflammation [Videos 4 and 5].

MODIFICATIONS

The hairline brow lift is dissected in one of three different planes: subcutaneous, subgaleal, or subperiosteal. Most commonly the operation is carried out in the subcutaneous plane. This plane minimizes risk of permanent nerve damage and protects the deep branch of the supraorbital nerve, which is one of the most common reasons for postoperative hypoesthesia or worse chronic scalp pruritus in the brow lift patient.

The most common modification of this procedure is forehead reduction procedures. This requires a subgaleal dissection posteriorly beyond the scalp vertex. Scalp advancement can be augmented with galeal release through radial scoring perpendicular to the desired vector of scalp advancement. This procedure is often combined with bony anchoring to maintain new lower hairline position.

Hairline brow lifts can also be an effective tool in the armamentarium of gender reassignment surgery. This approach not only allows the modification of the brow position to a more gender appropriate position (ie, creating laterally elevated or peaked appearance in male to female patients), but by altering the plane of dissection can allow for simultaneous frontal bone and orbital rim modification. This is achieved by either transitioning initial subcutaneous or subgaleal dissection to subperiosteal in the caudal portion of the forehead a few centimeters above the supraorbital rim. An example of hairline brow lift technique combined with frontal and supraorbital bony contouring in a male to female gender reassignment patient is seen in **Fig. 9**.

Similarly, in patients requiring glabellar rejuvenation, the subcutaneous dissection is transitioned from superficial to deep to frontalis muscle in the medial forehead to expose corrugator and procerus musculature for resection.

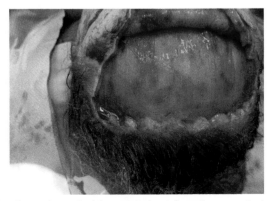

Fig. 8. Subcutaneous dissection from zigzag incision carried out from 2 mm posterior to anterior hairline to brow. Frontalis is maintained by direct visualization during dissection.

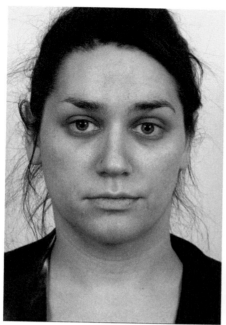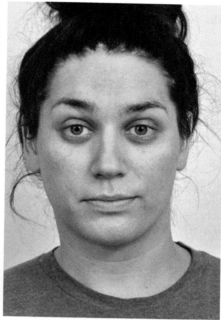

Fig. 9. Before (*left*) and after (*right*) of male to female gender reassignment patient 2 years after hairline brow lift performed in combination with bony contouring of frontal and supraorbital bones, anterior lipectomy and platysmaplasty, and genioplasty. Hairline brow lift was performed in subgaleal plane and transitioned to subperiosteal 2 cm above supraorbital rim for bony exposure.

CONCLUSION

The hairline incision brow lift remains an effective tool for addressing medial and lateral brow ptosis. This approach has the distinct advantages of preserving scalp sensation by protecting the deep branch of the supraorbital nerve, excellent exposure to frontalis and glabellar muscles for forehead rhytidectomy, potential for shortening of forehead in patients with high hairlines, minimization of postoperative alopecia, and shorter operative times because of ease of dissection.

It is critically important to evaluate patients for the presence of medial brow ptosis before surgery. Aging patients often present with lateral brow ptosis in the absence of concurrent medial brow position change and may be better suited for more limited incisions, such as temporal brow lifts. Preoperative discussion of postoperative scar appearance and placement is also important, because one of the biggest critiques of this procedure has been the long-standing scar appearance present in the anterior hairline. Despite these limitations, pretrichial approach to brow lift is a powerful procedure in appropriate patients because of its effective brow elevation and forehead rejuvenation, technical ease, and versatility in upper third facial rejuvenation. Finally it should be emphasized that successful correction of aging in the upper third of the face is not predicated on elevation of the brow alone, but rather on the combination of proper brow position combined with maintenance of improvement of brow shape. Thus today brow lifting is perhaps a misnomer and is better described as "brow shaping."

CLINICS CARE POINTS

- Hairline brow lifts candidates ideally are those with high hairlines and long foreheads.
- Advantages of hairline brow lifts are decreased injury risk to deep branch of supraorbital nerve, decreased risk of alopecia, addresses global brow ptosis, and decreased operative time because of ease of dissection.
- Hairline brow lifts should be avoided in patients with concern for postoperative scar appearance.
- Hairline brow lifts are easily modified for exposure to glabellar region for corrugator and procerus resection, hairline lowering with patients with long foreheads, and gender reassignment patients for exposure for bony contouring of frontal and supraorbital bossing.
- Patients with isolated lateral brow ptosis may be better served by more limited incisions, such as temporal brow lift.

DISCLOSURE

All authors have no conflicts of interest or sources of funding to disclose.

SUPPLEMENTARY DATA

Supplementary data to this article can be found online at https://doi.org/10.1016/j.cps.2022.01.004.

REFERENCES

1. Pitanguy I. Indications for and treatment of frontal and glabellar wrinkles in an analysis of 3,404 consecutive cases of rhytidectomy. Plast Reconstr Surg 1981;67(2):157–68.
2. Kaye BL. The forehead lift: a useful adjunct to face lift and blepharoplasty. Plast Reconstr Surg 1977; 60(2):161–71.
3. Guyuron B, Davies B. Subcutaneous anterior hairline forehead rhytidectomy. Aesthetic Plast Surg 1988; 12(2):77–83.
4. Pelle-Ceravolo M, Angelini M. Transcutaneous brow shaping: a straightforward and precise method to lift and shape eyebrows. Aesthet Surg J 2017;37(8):867–75.
5. Gleason MC. Brow lifting through a temporal scalp approach. Plast Reconstr Surg 1973;52(2):141–4.
6. Rohrich RJ, Beran SJ. Evolving fixation methods in endoscopically assisted forehead rejuvenation: controversies and rationale. Plast Reconstr Surg 1997; 100(6):1575–82.
7. Hunt HL. Plastic surgery of the head, face and neck. Lea & Febiger; 1926.
8. Miller TA, Rudkin G, Honig J, et al. Lateral subcutaneous brow lift and interbrow muscle resection:

9. clinical experience and anatomic studies. Plast Reconstr Surg 2000;105:1120–7.
9. Guyuron B, Belmand RA, Green R. Shortening the long forehead. Plast Reconstr Surg 1990;103:218–23.
10. Marten T. Hairline lowering during foreheadplasty. Plast Reconstr Surg 1999;103:224–36.
11. Yaremchuk MJ, O'Sullivan N, Benslimane F. Reversing brow lifts. Aesthet Surg J 2007;27:367–75.
12. Guyuron B, Lee M. A reappraisal of surgical techniques and efficacy in forehead rejuvenation. Plast Reconstr Surg 2014;134(3):426–35.
13. Connell BF, Lambros VS, Neurohr GH. The forehead lift: techniques to avoid complications and produce optimal results. Aesthetic Plast Surg 1989;13:217–37.
14. Stanley Klatsky MD, Robert W, Bernard MD, Bruce F, et al. The difficult forehead. Aesthet Surg J 2004; 24(2):146–54.
15. Camirand A, Doucet Jocelyne IL. A comparison between parallel hairline incisions and perpendicular incisions when performing a face lift. Plast Reconstr Surg 1997;99(1):10–5.
16. Cuoto RA, Charafeddine A, Sinclair NR, et al. Local infiltration of tranexamic acid with local anesthetic reduces intraoperative facelift bleeding: a preliminary report. Aesthet Surg J 2020;40(6):587–93.
17. Zins JE, Moreira-Gonzalez A. Cosmetic procedures for the aging face. Clin Geriatr Med 2006;22(3):709–28.
18. Zins Face Lift Marker [Internet]. Surgical instruments. Available at: http://www.accuratesurgical.com/products/forceps/product/3331-zins-face-lift-marker. Accessed January 11, 2022.

Endoscopic Brow Lift

James E. Zins, MD, FACS[a],*, Demetrius M. Coombs, MD[b]

KEYWORDS

- Endoscopic brow lift • Ptosis • Facial rejuvenation

KEY POINTS

- Description of the physiology of brow ptosis.
- Mechanism of endoscopic correction of brow ptosis.
- Detailed description of surgical technique.
- Pitfalls and flaws in endoscopic technique leading to adverse outcomes.

Video content accompanies this article at http://www.plasticsurgery.theclinics.com.

INTRODUCTION

Before 1991, the coronal brow lift was the gold standard for the correction of brow ptosis. However, the operation was not without postoperative complications and adverse sequelae including long-term numbness, pruritis, alopecia of the scalp, and scar deformity.[1]

Vasconez and Isse independently introduced the endoscopic brow lift in the early 1990s. Vasconez's approach was a subgaleal one. Isse's procedure highlighted depressor muscle alteration to gain the surgical result.[2–4]

After the introduction of the endoscopic brow, the initial enthusiasm was followed by a more recent decrease in the number of endoscopic procedures performed. The reasons for this were multifactorial. They included reports of dissatisfaction with the results, the quality and longevity of the operation, as well as the emergence of less technically challenging procedures such as the isolated temporal lift, the transpalpebral corrugator resection, and the so-called chemical brow lift using botulinum toxin.[5–10]

TECHNICAL ASPECTS

1. Over elevation of the brow

It is very easy to over elevate the medial brow using the endoscopic technique and it is very easy to place the lateral brow too low. The solution to over elevation of the medial brow is to preserve at least 2 cm of periosteal attachments in the midline glabellar region. The solution to obtaining adequate lateral brow elevation is wide subperiosteal release, which includes release of the superior temporal line, the temporal ligamentous adhesion, and the lateral orbital rim as far as the zygomatic arch.

2. The surprised look

With aging of the upper face, the medial brow often elevates due to static frontalis activation, whereas the lateral brow descends often below the level of the medial brow due to the lack of presence of elevator muscle laterally. This results in hooding of the brow laterally. Over elevation of the medial brow may lead to the so-called surprised look and is harmful to brow esthetics. However, even when over elevated, if brow shape is maintained, over elevation is relatively well tolerated. This highlights the modern dictum of upper face esthetics, which emphasizes maintenance or improvement of brow shape is more important than brow elevation (**Fig. 1**).

[a] Section of Cosmetic Surgery, Cleveland Clinic Department of Plastic Surgery, Desk A 60, 9500 Euclid Avenue, Cleveland, OH 44195, USA; [b] Cleveland Clinic Department of Plastic Surgery, Desk A 60, 9500 Euclid Avenue, Cleveland, OH 44195, USA
* Corresponding author.
E-mail address: zinsj@ccf.org

Clin Plastic Surg 49 (2022) 357–363
https://doi.org/10.1016/j.cps.2022.02.003
0094-1298/22/© 2022 Elsevier Inc. All rights reserved.

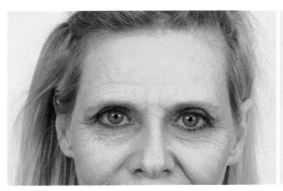 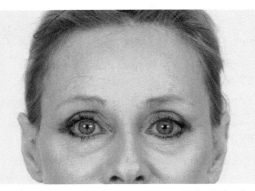

Fig. 1. Clinical photographs of a 61-year-old female Fitzpatrick I patient with brow ptosis and a high forehead who presented for facial rejuvenation (*left*). The same patient 3 months postoperatively following extended SMAS facelift and endoscopic brow lift using cortical tunnel technique for bony fixation of superficial temporal fascia to deep temporal fascia for temporal fixation (*right*). The early postoperative view shows over-correction and a surprised look.

PHYSIOLOGY OF BROW CORRECTION

The endoscopic brow lift gains its effect from a very different mechanism than the open coronal lift. The coronal brow lift owes its effect to a purely mechanical mechanism. As a general rule, 2.5 cm of scalp excision results in 1 cm of brow elevation. The endoscopic brow lift, on the other hand, owes its efficacy to an interplay between the elevators and depressor muscles of the forehead. When the depressors of the brow are weakened, the elevators work relatively unopposed.[4,11,12] This is combined with wide subperiosteal release of the superior temporal line, the temporal ligamentous adhesion, and the lateral orbital periosteum (**Fig. 2**). As no skin is excised in the forehead with the endoscopic brow lift, it is this alteration of muscles and periosteal release that gains the effect rather than mechanical pull.

LONGEVITY OF THE ENDOSCOPIC TECHNIQUE

Although some controversy remains regarding the long-term maintenance of the endoscopic brow, multiple studies document the statistically significant correction of brow ptosis long-term[13–17] (**Fig. 3**). More recently, however, it has become apparent that success in brow lifting should not be predicated on brow elevation alone but rather it should focus on maintaining or improving brow shape. The brow lift restores the loss of definition that occurs with aging. This loss of definition of the superior lateral supraorbital rim cannot be obtained by upper lid blepharoplasty alone (**Fig. 4**).

ANATOMY

Several critical structures require highlighting along the lateral aspect of the supraorbital rim,

there is a broad retaining ligament or adhesion between the galea and periosteum known as the temporal ligamentous adhesion. This along with the superior temporal line or septum and the supraorbital ligamentous adhesion need to be released subperiosteally to gain lateral brow elevation.

The inferior temporal septum runs from the superior lateral orbital rim to the posterior zygomatic arch. Above this line, there are no important structures. Below this line lie the sentinel vein and the frontal branch of the facial nerve. The sentinel vein lies 1 cm lateral and superior to the lateral canthus. The frontal branch lies 1 cm superior and lateral to the vein. Therefore, once the vein has been visualized, the frontal branch has been passed (see **Fig. 2**).

TECHNIQUE

The key to success with regard to technique is maintaining the proper anatomic planes. This means dissecting on the deep temporal fascia and the superficial layer of the deep temporal fascia in the temple to the lateral orbital rim laterally and subperiosteally at the level of the superior lateral and lateral orbital rim medially.

Operative Steps

1. Five incisions are made. One incision is made in the right and one incision in the left temple on a line from the alar base through the lateral canthus. Three or 4 incisions are made in the scalp several centimeters into the hairline. One incision is made in the right and one incision in the left lateral forehead scalp on a vertical line from the lateral third of the brow. One incision is then made in the midline of the

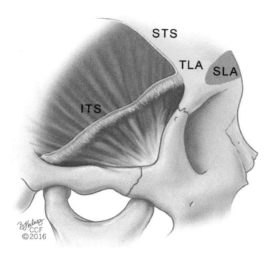

Fig. 2. Anatomic illustration of lateral brow structures including the inferior temporal septum (ITS), superior temporal septum (STS), temporal ligamentous adhesion (TLA), and supraorbital ligamentous adhesion (SLA). (*Courtesy of* Cleveland Clinic Center for Medical Art & Photography, Cleveland, OH.). (Reprinted with permission, Cleveland Clinic Foundation 2022. All Rights Reserved.)

forehead scalp skin or alternatively 2 paramedian incisions are made (**Fig. 5**).

2. The temporal incision is made first. Dissection is taken through the superficial temporal fascia in the deep temporal fascia. Deep temporal fascia is clearly recognized as pure white. The superior temporal line is then released posterior to anterior. It is important to dissect subperiosteally immediately medial to the superior temporal line as the deep branch of the supraorbital nerve lies 1 to 2 cm medial to the line between periosteum and galea. Injury to this nerve can result in numbness or pruritis of the scalp postoperatively. The temporal ligamentous adhesion and the lateral orbital rim are then released subperiosteally into the midface. This allows for not only brow release but also improvement in the midface. As all lateral soft tissue structures are thus released except for the deep head of the lateral canthal tendon, this results in a canthopexy type effect (Video 1).

3. Forehead dissection

The forehead is released subperiosteally through the 3 to 4 forehead incisions sequentially. The subperiosteal release extends down to the supraorbital rims. Two centimeters of periosteal attachment is spared medially at the glabella to prevent over elevation of the medial brow. The

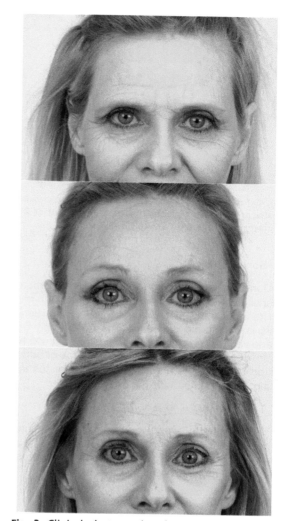

Fig. 3. Clinical photographs of a 61-year-old female Fitzpatrick I patient with brow ptosis and a high forehead who presented for facial rejuvenation (*left*). The same patient 3 months postoperatively following extended SMAS facelift and endoscopic brow lift using cortical tunnel technique for bony fixation of superficial temporal fascia to deep temporal fascia for temporal fixation; the early postoperative view shows over-correction and a surprised look (*center*). The same patient now 68 years old and nearly 7 years postoperatively; long-term follow-up demonstrates stability of the results (*right*).

arcus marginalis is released in its entirety. The step creates brow elevation (Video 2).

4. Corrugator and procerus resection

The corrugator muscles and if indicated the procerus are resected. The end point of corrugator resection is skeletonization of the supraorbital nerves and visualization of subcutaneous fat (**Fig. 6**).

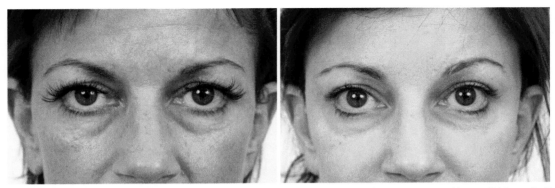

Fig. 4. Preoperative photograph of a 51-year-old woman with facial aging, brow ptosis, and lower lid bags (*left*). Postoperative photographs of the same patient at 2 years following endoscopic brow lift, lower eyelid blepharoplasty, and extended SMAS facelift.

5. Bone fixation

Bone fixation is accomplished using the cortical tunnel technique. The tunnel is placed through the posterior aspect of the lateral forehead incision. This is very rapid and safe. The tunnel can be made very superficially. A bone cut approximately 2 mm deep with a very narrow bone bridge or bone island between the anterior and posterior tunnel using a side cutting burr (Video 3).

6. Tail of the brow elevation

This is accomplished by suturing the superficial temporal fascia to the deep temporal fascia in a superior and posterior direction with 1-2 sutures of 2-0 PDS (polydioxanone) suture (Video 4).

ALTERNATIVE MEANS OF FIXATION

A variety of other devices have been used for fixation purposes in addition to the cortical tunnel. This includes Endotines, Mitek suture anchors, and fibrin glue. The literature supports superior fixation with the cortical tunnel technique when compared with fibrin glue.[11] When using the cortical tunnel, Jones and Grover found that permanent sutures were more effective than absorbable sutures with regard to longevity. Finally, multiple authors maintain that broad subperiosteal release is more important with regard to correction than bone fixation. In fact, several authors question the need for bone fixation at all and have demonstrated similar results with and without bony fixation.[15–17]

PATIENT SELECTION

The best candidates for endo brow lift are those with short or normal forehead height, a flat forehead, and those with no receding hairline and minimal true medial skin excess. Conversely, poor candidates are those with a convex forehead,

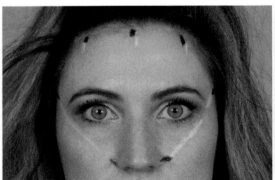
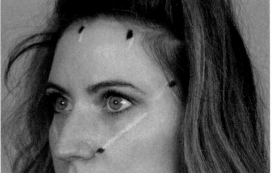

Fig. 5. Clinical photographs depicting the incisions for endoscopic brow lift. The temporal incision is made on a line drawn from the alar base to the lateral canthus within the temporal hairline. The lateral forehead incision is made on a vertical line from the lateral two-thirds of the brow to correspond to the apex of the brow. The medial incision is for access to the corrugator/procerus muscles. Please note that the incisions are made within the hairline. Marks on the skin are for demonstrative purposes only.

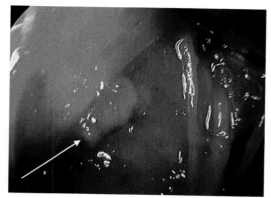

Fig. 6. Intraoperative endoscopic view of a partially resected left corrugator muscle (denoted by the *white arrow*) with supratrochlear branches skeletonized (right aspect of the image).

high hairline, deep rhytids, thick skin, and true medial skin excess (**Fig. 7**).

TRAPS AND FLAWS

1. Early recurrence of glabellar lines

This occurs because of inadequate glabellar muscle removal and is prevented by the removal of all muscle between bone and subcutaneous fat.

2. Asymmetry

True asymmetry needs to be differentiated from asymmetry due to upper eyelid ptosis. True asymmetry is structural and should be noted preoperatively. Differential fixation is indicated. It is a reasonable rule of thumb to mention to the patient that if there is asymmetry preoperatively, there may be some degree postoperatively as well. This true asymmetry should be differentiated

from asymmetry due to frontalis activation due to unilateral upper eyelid ptosis. Patients with asymmetry due to unilateral upper eyelid ptosis will often have a high supratarsal fold and crease. In such cases, upper eyelid ptosis repair is indicated.

3. Over elevation

The surprised look results from a combination of overly aggressive medial subperiosteal release, release of the medial depressors, and/or overly aggressive lateral brow elevation. If noted, early fixation can be adjusted.

4. Under elevation of the lateral brow

Inadequate lateral brow elevation results from insufficient subperiosteal release and requires reoperation if significant.

5. Displeasing eyebrow arch

Unattractive brow shape is generally due to excessive medial brow subperiosteal release and inadequate lateral release.

QUALITY OF STUDIES

There are no prospective randomized studies comparing open and endoscopic techniques. Further few studies have compared long-term outcomes of the 2 techniques in detail. Finally, few studies use validated subjective and objective grading systems to assess brow shape long-term.[17–19]

The best study addressing long-term results in endoscopic brow lifting using validated tools was the Jones and Lo report.[19] They found statistically significant brow elevation of 3.5 to 4.7 mm at all 5 points measured medial to lateral across the up to 1 year. At 5 years, statistically significant elevation

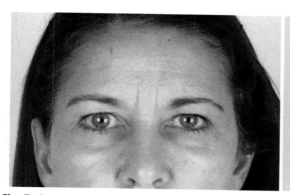
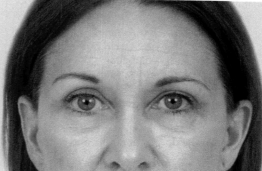

Fig. 7. Preoperative photographs of a 63-year-old female with brow ptosis, corrugator hyperactivity, and deep nasolabial folds presenting for facial rejuvenation (*left*). The same patient 14 months postoperatively following facelift, endoscopic brow lift with complete corrugator resection, bone fixation using cortical tunnels, and fixation of the superficial temporal fascia to the deep temporal fascia laterally.

was found at all 5 points again except for the most lateral point on the brow (brow tail). This point had reverted to preoperative baseline. Furthermore, the highest point of the brow was at the medial limbus rather than the lateral limbus. The authors hypothesized that the temporal fixation of superficial temporal fascia to deep temporal fascia was not strong enough to overcome the depressor effect of the lateral orbicularis oculi.

SUMMARY

Success in modern brow lifting surgery is predicated not on brow elevation alone but rather on improving or maintaining brow shape. Therefore, perhaps the term brow lift is a misnomer and the term used should be brow contouring. Technically medial brow elevation should be avoided. Lateral brow elevation requires wide subperiosteal release including the superior temporal line, the temporal ligamentous adhesion, and the lateral orbital rim to the zygomatic arch and into the midface.

Although the amount of elevation is not great, as documented by Jones and Lo, it is enough for consistent subjective improvement according to validated measures.

CLINICS CARE POINTS

- Unlike the coronal brow lift that depends on a pure mechanical pull, success in endoscopic brow lifting depends on weakening of the depressor muscles of the brow and wide subperiosteal undermining of the superior temporal line, the temporal ligamentous adhesion, and subperiosteal release of the lateral orbital rim to the zygomatic arch.

- It is very easy to over elevate the medial brow and easy to under elevate the lateral brow.

- Over elevation of the medial brow is prevented by leaving 2 cm of periosteum attached at the glabellar midline. Under elevation laterally is prevented by wide subperiosteal undermining.

- The key to success technically is remaining in the correct plane. That is on top of the deep temporal fascia and superficial layer of the deep temporal fascia laterally and subperiosteal medially.

- Successful brow lift surgery is not predicated on brow elevation but rather on maintaining or improving brow shape. Perhaps brow shaping rather than lifting is a more accurate term.

DISCLOSURE

All authors have nothing to disclose.

SUPPLEMENTARY DATA

Supplementary data related to this article can be found online at https://doi.org/10.1016/j.cps.2022.02.003.

REFERENCES

1. Paul MD. The evolution of the brow lift in aesthetic plastic surgery. Plast Reconstr Surg 2001;108:1409–24.
2. Isse NG. Endoscopic facial rejuvenation: endoforehead, the functional lift. case reports. Aesthet Plast Surg 1994;18:21–9.
3. Vasconez LO. The use of the Endoscope in brow lifting. Washington, DC: Annual Meeting 7of the American Society of Plastic and Reconstructive Surgeons; 1992. Video presentation at.
4. Isse NG. Endoscopic forehead lift: evolution and update. Clin Plast Surg 1995;22:661.
5. Chiu ES, Baker DC. Endoscopic brow lift: a retrospective review of 628 consecutive cases over 5 years. Plast Reconstr Surg 2003;112:628–33. ; discussion 634-635.
6. Tabatabai N, Spinelli HM. Limited incision nonendoscopic brow lift. Plast Reconstr Surg 2007;119:1563–70.
7. Rohrich RJ, Cho M-J. Endoscopic temporal brow lift: surgical indications, technique, and 10-year outcomes analysis. Plast Reconstr Surg 2019;144:1305–10.
8. Mass CS, Kim EJ. Temporal brow lift using botulinum toxin a: an update. Plast Reconstr Surg 2003;112(Suppl):109S–12S. ; discussion 113s-114S.
9. Kane MA. Nonsurgical periorbital and brow rejuvenation. Plas Reconstr Surg 2015;135:63–71.
10. Jones BM, Grover R. Endoscopic brow lift: a personal review of 538 patients and comparison of fixation techniques. Plast Reconstr Surg 2004;113:1242–50. Discussion 1251-1252.
11. Knize DM. Limited Incision forehead lift for eyebrow elevation to enhance upper lid blepharoplasty. Plast Reconstr Surg 2001;108:564–7.
12. Knize DM. An anatomically based study of the mechanism of eyebrow ptosis. Plast Reconstr Surg 1996;97(7):1321–33.
13. Guyuron BM. Endoscopic forehead rejuvenation: limitations, flaws and rewards. Plast Reconstr Surg 2006;117:1121–33.
14. Behmand RA. Guyuron BM Endoscopic forehead rejuvenation:11 Long-term results. Plast Reconstr Surg 2006;117:1137–43. Discussion 1144.
15. Troilius CA. A comparison between subgaleal and subperiosteal brow lifts. Plast Reconstr Surg 1999;104:1079–90. Discussion 1091-1092.

16. Guyuron BG, Kopal C, Michelow BJ. Stabilitiy after Endoscopic forehead surgery using single point fascia fixation. Plast Reconstr Surg 2005;116:1988–94.

17. Iblher N, Manegold S, Porzelius C. Morphometric Long term evaluation and comparison of brow position and shape after Endoforehead lift and transpalpebral Browpexy. Plast Reconstr Surg 2012;130:830e–40e.

18. Graham DW, Heller J, Kirkjian TJ, et al. Brow lift in facial rejuvenation: a systemic literature review of open versus endoscopic techniques. Plast Reconstr Surg 2011;128:335e–41e.

19. Jones BM, Lo SJ. The Impact of endoscopic brow lift on eyebrow morphology, aesthetics, and longevity: objective and subjective measurements over a 5 year period. Plast Reconstr Surg 2013;132:226e–38e.

Subcutaneous Lateral Temporal Lift

Ira L. Savetsky, MD[a], Joshua M. Cohen, MD[b], Alan Matarasso, MD[c],*

KEYWORDS

- Brow lift - Lateral temporal lift - Subcutaneous temporal lift - Subcutaneous brow lift - Brow ptosis
- Brow rejuvenation - Forehead rejuvenation

KEY POINTS

- An in-depth understanding of forehead anatomy and natural aging allows for effective preoperative analysis and subsequent development of a patient-specific treatment plan.
- The subcutaneous temporal brow lift is a safe, effective, and reliable method for correction of lateral brow ptosis.
- Surgical markings should be performed with the patient in a seated upright position, and care should be taken when evaluating brow ptosis in the setting of chronic frontalis activation and dermatochalasis.

INTRODUCTION

Achieving the ideal aesthetic of the forehead and brow is a critical part of establishing facial harmony. The plastic surgery literature has traditionally focused on rejuvenation of the face and brow. However, interest in periorbital rejuvenation may have increased further because of mask wearing during the COVID-19 pandemic. An increased focus on periorbital aesthetics is logical because the eyes and eyebrows are the first part of the face that others notice, as well as the most expressive part of the face. The eyes have been called the window to the soul, whereas the brows are a curtain of emotion. The ability to express this range of emotions through one's eyes and eyebrows is an important form of nonverbal communication that helps cross language barriers and cultural differences. Although the unnaturally elevated brow can lead to the so-called surprised look, the aging forehead and brow can lead to the unintentional expression of sadness, anger, or fatigue.[1,2]

Various techniques have been established over the past 30 years to correct the aging brow, ranging from the least invasive, such as neurotoxin, to open surgical correction. The senior author has used multiple techniques for forehead rejuvenation, but his current preferred method is the lateral subcutaneous temporal lift, which is described in detail in later discussion.[3]

HISTORY OF FOREHEAD REJUVENATION

The evolution of forehead rejuvenation was well documented by Paul[4] in 2001 and begins with Passot in 1919. Passot's brow-lift technique involved multiple direct skin excisions above the eyebrow, hidden in forehead rhytids.[5] Although Passot only excised skin and subcutaneous tissue, others recommended inclusion of muscle. In 1926, Hunt[6] published the first description of an incision in the scalp or anterior hairline for brow lifting. Lexer and Lexer,[7] known for performing the first facelift, published their combined face and forehead lift procedure in 1931. The next major

[a] Private Practice, 6000 West Spring Creek, Suite 200, Plano, TX 75024, USA; [b] Hansjörg Wyss Department of Plastic Surgery, NewYork University Langone Health, 222 East 41st Street, New York, NY 10017, USA; [c] Northwell Health System/Hofstra University, Zucker School of Medicine, Manhattan Eye, Ear and Throat Hospital, 1009 Park Avenue, New York, NY 10028, USA
* Corresponding author.
E-mail address: amatarasso@drmatarasso.com
Twitter: @DrAlanMatarasso (A.M.)

Clin Plastic Surg 49 (2022) 365–375
https://doi.org/10.1016/j.cps.2022.02.001

advancement in forehead rejuvenation came in the 1960s when Vinas described the importance of lateral brow elevation in brow lift.[8] Advances continued to be made in the 1980s with Papillon's description of a subcutaneous plane of dissection and Paul's description of his transblepharoplasty approach.[9,10] In 1992, the endoscopic brow lift was first presented at meetings by Isse and Vasconez and subsequently published in the literature in 1993 by Chajchir.[11–13] Although the twenty-first century brings a renewal of various techniques and competing philosophies, the goal remains the same: correction of brow ptosis in a reproducible and long-term manner while maintaining or improving brow shape while causing minimal scarring, nerve injury, alopecia, and hairline distortion.

ANATOMY

An understanding of facial anatomy, surface landmarks, and natural aging is crucial when addressing rejuvenation of the upper one-third of the face.[14,15] The bony forehead is made up of the frontal bone, which is crossed laterally by the temporal ridge. The temporal ridge is critical, as all fascial layers are tethered to this "zone of fixation." Inferiorly, the attachments widen to become the orbital ligament. Lateral and inferior to this zone is the inferior temporal septum, which becomes a landmark for endoscopic forehead surgery because the frontal branch of the facial nerve and the sentinel vein are both inferior and medial to this attachment.[16] The lateral-most part of the superficial temporal fascia has attachments to the zone of fixation and weakens over time owing to the effects of gravity. As the superficial temporal fascia descends, so do overlying tissues, including the lateral brow, leading to the classic sad-appearing eyes. The medial brow continues to be supported by the frontalis muscle and the brow depressor muscles. Descent of the galeal fat pad can also contribute to lateral eyebrow ptosis.[17] Typically, the galeal fat pad is encompassed by layers of the galea. However, some patients have no galeal support inferior to the fat pad, which allows it to descend with age.

The level of the eyebrow is also intimately linked to the action of the surrounding muscles and the universal depressor: gravity. The frontalis muscle is the only elevator of the brow. It originates from the galea and interdigitates with the orbicularis oculi. The action of the frontalis leads to transverse forehead skin lines. There are multiple brow depressors that originate from the glabella and insert into the soft tissue. The procerus runs in a vertical fashion; the depressor supercilii and orbicularis run obliquely, and the corrugator runs transversely

and obliquely. These muscles create transverse, oblique, and vertical glabellar skin lines, respectively. As one ages, these skin lines deepen, and with continued actinic changes of the overlying skin and weakening of the underlying collagen, become apparent at rest. The lateral orbicularis oculi is the only lateral muscular depressor of the brow.[16]

The muscles of the forehead are controlled by the temporal branch of the facial nerve. The temporal branch crosses the middle third of the zygomatic arch in a supraperiosteal plane, deep to the parotid temporal fascia. It becomes more superficial approximately 2 cm above the arch, entering the superficial temporal fascia at this point. The temporal branch can be protected during forehead rejuvenation by either performing dissection directly on the deep temporal fascia in the temple, remaining deep to the superficial layer of the deep temporal fascia inferiorly, and in the subgaleal or subperiosteal plane over the frontal bone or performing dissection superficial to the superficial temporal fascia and the surrounding forehead muscles.[18] Another important landmark for the frontal branch is the sentinel vein, which travels 1 cm medial and superior to the nerve and should be protected during endoscopic forehead lifts. The supraorbital and supratrochlear nerves provide sensory innervation to the forehead and peribrow skin. The supraorbital nerve exits above the orbit in either the supraorbital notch or the foramen. The notch can sometimes be felt transcutaneously and falls approximately 2.5 cm from the midline. If the nerve exits a foramen, this has been found to be as much as 1.9 cm above the orbital rim. Because of this variable anatomy, blind dissection should not be performed within 2 cm of the orbital rim.[19] The supratrochlear nerve exits the orbit medial to the supraorbital nerve and immediately divides into multiple branches, which typically pass through the substance of the corrugator muscles. These nerves should both be safe during a lateral subcutaneous temporal lift, as they both will lay medial to the dissection.

Multiple studies have evaluated the change of brow height over time. Although it has been classically thought and logical that all eyebrows descend with time, there is evidence in the literature that some brows can elevate as we age. Lambros[14] evaluated the long-term effects of periorbital aging and observed that in his cohort brow position elevated in greater than one-fourth of patients, was stable in a little less than half, and descended in greater than one-fourth of patients.[20] Brow elevation is secondary to "spastic frontalis syndrome" as described by Ramirez,[21] a compensatory mechanism of frontalis contraction in an effort to relieve the lateral soft tissue hooding from a ptotic brow, or in an attempt to alleviated partial vision obstruction.

The ideal brow position, as described by West-more[22] in 1974, starts medially on the same vertical plane as the ala and medial canthus and ends laterally at an oblique line from the ala through the lateral canthus. The medial and lateral ends of the brow lie on the same horizontal plane, while the brow peaks on a vertical line directly above the lateral limbus or at the lateral third of the brow. The height of the "ideal" peak is typically higher in women than in men. A survey of plastic surgeons and cosmetologists on their preferences for female eyebrow shape and height determined that the medial brow should be about the level of the supraorbital rim and have an apex lateral cant. A common error seen in brow lifting is over-elevation of the medial brow and underelevation of the lateral brow. Although brow elevation may thus occur, overelevation of the medial brow leads to an unattractive appearance.[23,24]

PREOPERATIVE EVALUATION

Patients presenting for periorbital rejuvenation typically have one or more of the following complaints: forehead and/or glabellar lines, a sad or heavy appearance to the eyes, drooping eyelids and/or eyebrows, bulges, or partially obstructed vision. Although the original option for treatment of the forehead was the classic coronal incision or direct brow lift, several more recent means of treating the aging forehead have generally replaced these techniques.[25] However, with advances comes the need for in-depth facial analysis.

The entire face should first be globally examined for symmetry and signs of aging. The patient can be asked to bring an old photograph to determine the predominant changes and to highlight areas of possible improvement. Next, the upper one-third of the face is evaluated as a unit. This evaluation begins with the patient sitting upright and looking forward in neutral gaze. An assessment should made of the patient's visual acuity, eyebrow/orbit relationship and symmetry, eyebrow shape and axis, eyebrow mobility, and forehead and glabellar rhytids. The patient should be evaluated with their eyes both closed and open. By having the patient close their eyes, the frontalis muscle relaxes as the ptotic lateral brow tissue is no longer causing partial vision obstruction. The location of the resting brow is noted, and the surgeon can manually reposition the brow to the ideal location. The eyelid is then evaluated for dermatochalasis, and an elevation test (**Fig. 1**) is performed to verify whether a

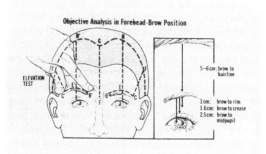

Fig. 1. The elevation test. The brow is manually elevated to the desired normal position. If there is any excess upper eyelid skin, an upper blepharoplasty may be indicated. (*Courtesy of* Alan Matarasso, MD, New York, NY.)

concurrent blepharoplasty and ptosis repair are needed.

MANAGEMENT OF FOREHEAD AGING

There is a wide range of options for management of forehead aging. The mainstay of treatment for dynamic forehead rhytids and glabellar creases is neurotoxin. Neurotoxin blocks nerves from releasing acetylcholine, thereby preventing contraction of the target muscle. The current neurotoxins in use are based on botulinum toxin serotype A and include Botox (onabotulinumtoxin A; Dublin, Ireland), Dysport (abobotulinumtoxin A; Galderma, Lausanne, Switzerland), and Xeomin (incobotulinumtoxin A, Merz, Frankfurt, Germany). Although there are recommended doses of injection depending on the location, the effect of botulinum toxin can range from a softening of dynamic rhytids during expression to complete paralysis of the target muscle leading to a "frozen" appearance. Ultimately, facial analysis, patient expectations, experience, and goals dictate the endpoint. Static rhytids can be best treated by laser resurfacing and chemical peels.

Although neurotoxin can be used to minimally "lift" the brow with denervation of the eyebrow depressors and preservation of the lower frontalis muscle (therefore also leaving those lower rhytids), brow ptosis is best treated with surgical intervention. The open-coronal approach, once deemed the "gold standard," is a good option for forehead rejuvenation with wide surgical exposure and the ability to effectively mobilize brow tissues and modify muscle attachments under direct visualization. Incisions can either be camouflaged in the hair-bearing scalp or be along the anterior hairline in the long forehead. As the anterior hairline avoids undermining of hair follicles, the plane of dissection can be as superficial as the subcutaneous plane above the frontalis. This allows for safe and efficient brow elevation and potential effacement of rhytids without concern for transection of major neurovascular structures. The endoscopic brow lift was the next major advancement and was able to address many of the same issues dealt with by open coronal brow lift, however with reduced scar burden, postoperative edema, and risk of nerve injury.[3] With the endoscopic approach, it is very easy to overelevate the medial brow and difficult to adequately elevate the lateral brow.

The senior author began performing lateral temporal brow lifts in the early 2000s, first dissecting in the subperiosteal plane, then biplanar, and finally only subcutaneously. The benefits of the subcutaneous lateral temporal lift are numerous and include safe, repeatable, and effective elevation of the lateral brow.

SUBCUTANEOUS LATERAL TEMPORAL LIFT
Preoperative Markings

Appropriate preoperative markings guide the surgeon in providing a symmetric brow lift and appropriate forehead height. All markings are performed with the patient seated upright. The patient is first asked to relax their forehead, and then the midline of the forehead (widow's peak in select patients) is marked. The ellipse begins approximately 3.5 cm lateral from midline, which corresponds to about the midpupillary line. The ellipse is marked to be 4 to 5 cm in length and 2 to 2.5 cm in width depending on the amount of brow lift needed. The width is narrower in patients with a less ptotic brow and narrower forehead. The axis of the ellipse typically runs parallel to the brow.

The incision can be placed either in the hair-bearing scalp or at the hairline (**Fig. 2**). A hairline incision would allow for the height of the forehead to be reduced. Additional thought must be taken for patients who have thin hair density and who are less likely to hide a hair-bearing scalp incision. However, if the incision is carefully made in the orientation of hair follicle growth, the incision can be well concealed.

Surgical Technique

The patient's hair is combed back and wrapped in a blue towel. The operative field is prepared, and the marked incisions are infiltrated with approximately 20 mL of 0.5% lidocaine with epinephrine at 1:200,000. Once adequate anesthesia has been achieved, the ellipse of skin is excised down to the subcutaneous tissue. The inferior dissection begins sharply with a no. 10 blade just

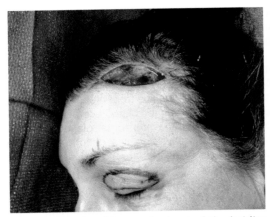

Fig. 2. A typical incision at the level of the hairline, which begins at the midpupillary line and extends 5 cm in length. (*Courtesy of* Alan Matarasso, MD, New York, NY.)

above the frontalis muscle. Once the appropriate plane has been developed, blunt finger dissection ensues inferiorly, medially, and laterally. Any residual points of adhesion are taken down with a face-lift scissors until the upper edge of the eyebrow is reached. The dissection is slightly wider than the width of the initial ellipse to allow for appropriate elevation of the eyebrow and effective redraping of the forehead skin (**Fig. 3**). Hemostasis is

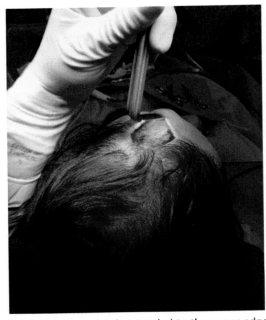

Fig. 3. The dissection is extended to the upper edge of the eyebrow and is wider than the length of the incision. (*Courtesy of* Alan Matarasso, MD, New York, NY.)

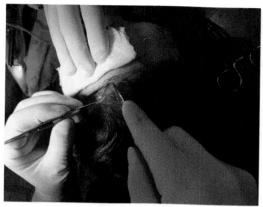

Fig. 4. Before closure, a fibrin sealant is applied to the wound bed, and pressure is held for 3 minutes. (*Courtesy of* Alan Matarasso, MD, New York, NY.)

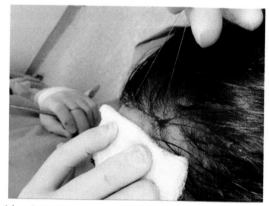

Fig. 5. The wound is closed with a 3-0 Monoderm bidirectional Quill suture (Surgical Specialties Corp). (*Courtesy of* Alan Matarasso, MD, New York, NY.)

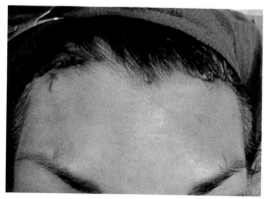

Fig. 6. Appearance of the on-table result after closure of the incision. (*Courtesy of* Alan Matarasso, MD, New York, NY.)

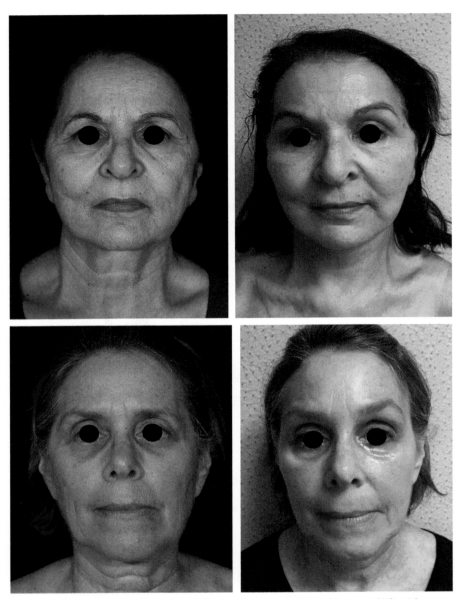

Fig. 7. Two patients who underwent the senior author's subcutaneous lateral temporal lift with preoperative and postoperative images. (*Courtesy of* Alan Matarasso, MD, New York, NY.)

achieved on the first side, and a sponge with 0.5% lidocaine with epinephrine at 1:200,000 is packed into the wound. This is repeated on the contralateral side. Attention is then turned back to the first side to achieve a final round of hemostasis. Fibrin sealant is used in the wound, and 3 minutes of pressure is applied on the forehead skin to allow for hemostatic curing of the sealant (**Fig. 4**). The wound is closed with a 3-0 Monoderm bidirectional Quill suture (Surgical Specialties Corp, Tijuana, Mexico) with a diamond point needle (**Fig. 5**). Interrupted 5-0 Prolene sutures (Ethicon, New Brunswick, NJ, USA) are used to decrease any tension on the incision (**Fig. 6**). The incisions are not dressed, and Prolene sutures can be removed in 3 to 5 days.

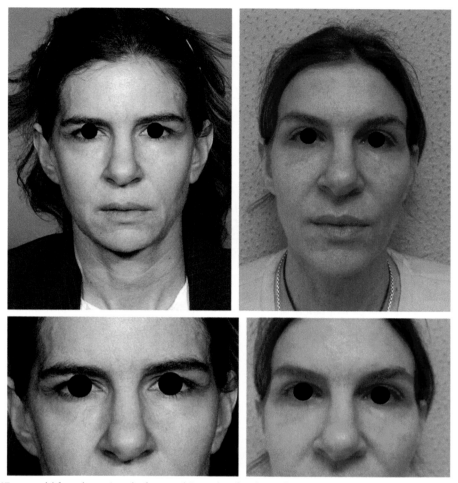

Fig. 8:. A 47-year-old female patient before and 6 weeks after lateral temporal browlift, upper lid blepharoplasty, and periocular erbium laser. (*Courtesy of* Alan Matarasso, MD, New York, NY.)

Expected Outcomes and Complications

The subcutaneous lateral temporal lift is a well-tolerated procedure with very few significant postoperative complications. The senior author published a retrospective review of his 500 consecutive subcutaneous lateral temporal lifts and found no cases of permanent nerve injury or skin necrosis. Patients were uniformly pleased with their postoperative results (**Figs. 7–12**). Of the 500 cases, there were a total of 3 hematomas/seromas, which were aspirated, and 2 cases of incisional alopecia and unsatisfactory scarring, requiring scar revision.[26]

A systematic review of the literature found 5 other retrospective studies that evaluated postoperative results following subcutaneous lateral brow lifts.[26] Miller and colleagues[27] reported their positive experience with the procedure in 65 patients. All patients had improvement in their brow ptosis and also in their hairline owing to excision of a triangular area of thinning hair in the temporal area. Miller also performed direct excision of glabellar facial muscles to decrease vertical rhytids. There were no episodes of permanent diminished scalp sensation or alopecia after the procedure. Bernard and colleagues[28] reported their experience with the procedure in 117 patients

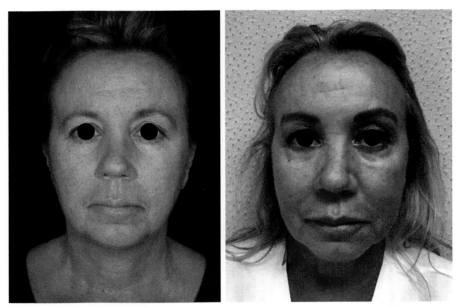

Fig. 9. A 55-year-old female patient before and 5 years after temporal browlift, upper lid blepharoplasty, and periocular erbium laser. (*Courtesy of* Alan Matarasso, MD, New York, NY.)

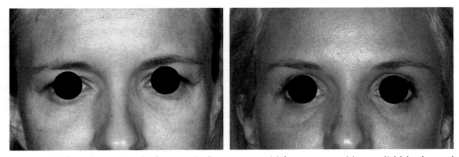

Fig. 10. A 42-year-old female patient before and after temporal lift, upper and lower lid blepharoplasty. (*Courtesy of* Alan Matarasso, MD, New York, NY.)

A

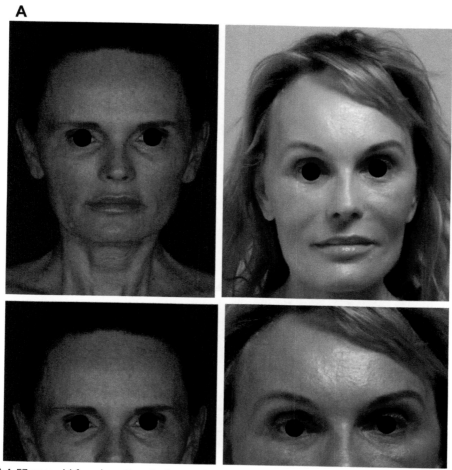

Fig. 11. (*A*) A 57-year-old female patient before and 1 month after lateral temporal lift. (*B*) Same 57-year-old female patient before and 5 years after lateral temporal lift. (*Courtesy of* Alan Matarasso, MD, New York, NY.)

over a 2-year period. The average operative time for the bilateral procedure was 23 minutes. Two patients developed hematomas, which required evacuation, and no patients had long-standing scalp hypesthesia or alopecia. Guerrissi[29] used a subcutaneous technique in conjunction with deep structure suspension to the temporal aponeurosis in 142 patients from 1999 to 2006. Although 91% of his patients had satisfactory results, 16% of patients developed "partial infection" of the temporal wound, and 9% of patients had immediate asymmetry of their eyebrows. In 2010, Bidros and colleagues[30] reported their results on 28 patients, almost all of whom rated their results as "good" or "excellent" with no incidences of hematoma, infection, hypesthesia, or poor scarring. Mahmood and Baker[31] reported durable results with no complications in their cohort of 100 patients.

SUMMARY

With in-depth preoperative planning and precise surgical technique, the subcutaneous temporal brow lift is a reliable and safe option for lateral brow elevation. The advantages of a subcutaneous dissection are numerous, including its safety, shorter operative time, feasibility under local anesthesia, and consistent long-term results with low likelihood of complications.

DISCLOSURE

The authors have no financial interest to disclose in relation to the content of this article.

B

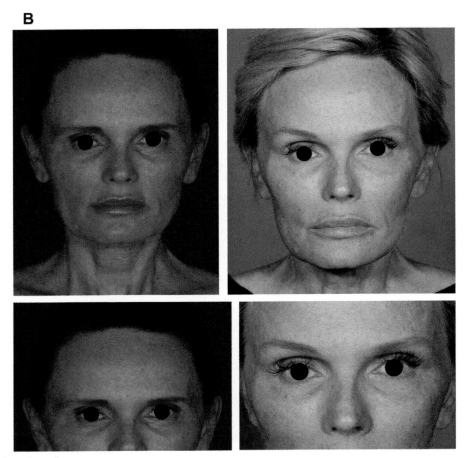

Fig. 11. (*continued*)

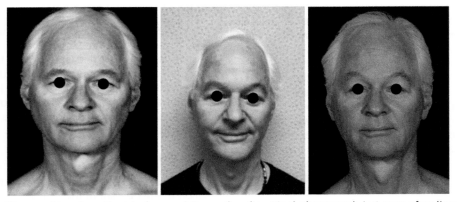

Fig. 12. A 69-year-old male patient before and 3 months after. Final photograph is 1 year after liposuction of abdomen, neck lift, mid-forehead browlift. Because of his hairline and the lengthy flap undermining required, a mid-forward incision was used. (*Courtesy of* Alan Matarasso, MD, New York, NY.)

CLINICS CARE POINTS

- An elevation test should be performed to verify whether the patient is a candidate for concurrent blepharoplasty with the temporal brow lift.

- Blind dissection of the forehead should not be performed within 2 cm of the orbital rim to protect the supraorbital nerve.

- Hemostasis should be checked multiple times before closure, and the addition of fibrin sealants can be used to decrease the most common complication of the procedure.

REFERENCES

1. Knoll BI, Attkiss KJ, Persing JA. The influence of forehead, brow, and periorbital aesthetics on perceived expression in the youthful face. Plast Reconstr Surg 2008;121(5).
2. Matarasso A, Terino EO. Forehead-brow rhytidoplasty: reassessing the goals. Plast Reconstr Surg 1994;93(7).
3. Matarasso A. Endoscopically assisted forehead-brow rhytidoplasty: theory and practice. Aesthetic Plast Surg 1995;19(2):141–7.
4. Paul MD. The evolution of the brow lift in aesthetic plastic surgery. Plast Reconstr Surg 2001;108(5).
5. Passot R. La chururgie esthetique dew rides du visage. Presse Med 1919;(27):258–60.
6. Hunt H. Plastic surgery of the head, face, and neck. Philadelphia, PA: Lea & Febiger; 1926.
7. Lexer E, Lexer E. Die Gesamte Wiederherstellungs-Chirurgie, 1 & 2. Leipzig: Jahann Ambrosius Barth; 1931.
8. Vinas JC, Caviglia C, Cortinas JL. Forehead rhytidoplasty and brow lifting. Plast Reconstr Surg 1976; 57(4):445–54.
9. Papillon J, Perras C, Tirkanits B. A comparative analysis of forehead lift techniques. Boston: Annual Meeting of the American Society for Aesthetic Plastic Surgery; 1984.
10. Paul MD. The surgical management of upper eyelid hooding. Aesthetic Plast Surg 1989;13(3):183–7.
11. Isse N. Endoscopic forehead lift. Los Angeles, CA: Annual Meeting of the Los Angeles County Society of Plastic Surgeons; 1992.
12. Vasconez L. The use of the endoscope in brow lifting. Washington, DC: Annual Meeting of the American Society of Plastic and Reconstructive Surgeons; 1992.
13. Chajchir A. Endoscopia en cirugia plastica y estetica. In: Gonzalez Montaner L, Huriado Hoyo E, Altman R, editors. El Libro de Oro en Homenaje al Doctor Carlos Reussi. Buenos Aires: Associacion Medica Argentina; 1993.
14. Lambros V. Observations on periorbital and midface aging. Plast Reconstr Surg 2007;120(5).
15. Gunter JP, Antrobus SD. Aesthetic analysis of the eyebrows. Plast Reconstr Surg 1997;99(7):1808–16.
16. Knize DM. Anatomic concepts for brow lift procedures. Plast Reconstr Surg 2009;124(6):2118–26.
17. Knize DM. Reassessment of the coronal incision and subgaleal dissection for foreheadplasty. Plast Reconstr Surg 1998;102(2):478–89.
18. Agarwal CA, Mendenhall SD 3rd, Foreman KB, et al. The course of the frontal branch of the facial nerve in relation to fascial planes: an anatomic study. Plast Reconstr Surg 2010;125(2):532–7.
19. Knize DM. A study of the supraorbital nerve. Plast Reconstr Surg 1995;96(3):564–9.
20. Matros E, Garcia JA, Yaremchuk MJ. Changes in eyebrow position and shape with aging. Plast Reconstr Surg 2009;124(4):1296–301.
21. Ramirez OM. Discussion: subperiosteal brow lifts without fixation. Plast Reconstr Surg 2004;114(6).
22. Westmore M. Facial cosmetics in conjunction with surgery. Vancouver, British Columbia, Canada: Aesthetic Plastic Surgical Society Meeting; 1974.
23. Freund RM, Nolan WB 3rd. Correlation between brow lift outcomes and aesthetic ideals for eyebrow height and shape in females. Plast Reconstr Surg 1996;97(7):1343–8.
24. Yaremchuk MJ, O'Sullivan N, Benslimane F. Reversing brow lifts. Aesthet Surg J 2007;27(4):367–75.
25. Matarasso A, Hutchinson O. Evaluating rejuvenation of the forehead and brow: an algorithm for selecting the appropriate technique. Plast Reconstr Surg 2000;106(3).
26. Savetsky IL, Matarasso A. Lateral temporal subcutaneous brow lift: clinical experience and systematic review of the literature. Plast Reconstr Surg – Glob Open 2020;8(4).
27. Miller TA, Rudkin G, Honig M, et al. Lateral subcutaneous brow lift and interbrow muscle resection: clinical experience and anatomic studies. Plast Reconstr Surg 2000;105(3).
28. Bernard RW, Greenwald JA, Beran SJ, et al. Enhancing upper lid aesthetics with the lateral subcutaneous brow lift. Aesthet Surg J 2006;26(1):19–23.
29. Guerrissi JO. Periorbital rejuvenation: a safe subcutaneous approach to forehead, eyebrow, and orbicularis oculis muscle mobilization. Aesthetic Plast Surg 2010;34(2):147–52.
30. Bidros RS, Salazar-Reyes H, Friedman JD. Subcutaneous temporal browlift under local anesthesia: a useful technique for periorbital rejuvenation. Aesthet Surg J 2010;30(6):783–8.
31. Mahmood U, Baker JL Jr. Lateral subcutaneous brow lift: updated technique. Aesthet Surg J 2015; 35(5):621–4.

The Gliding Brow Lift

Fabiola Aguilera, MD[a], James C. Grotting, MD[b],*

KEYWORDS

- Brow lift • Gliding brow lift • Subcutaneous brow lift • Hemostatic net

KEY POINTS

- Presenting gliding brow lift technique as an alternative to lift and shape the brow with 1 or 2 tiny incisions.
- Combination of temporal subcutaneous brow lifting with the use of hemostatic net led to the development of this technique in effort of simplifying prior described procedures.
- This technique can also be used to treat temporal "bunching" following facelifting.

Video content accompanies this article at http://www.plasticsurgery.theclinics.com.

INTRODUCTION

Brow lift plays an important role in facial rejuvenation, especially when treating the upper third of the face. It is not uncommon to see patients in consultation inquiring about a blepharoplasty to achieve a more youthful appearance of the orbital region. However, when demonstrating their desired appearance, they elevate the tail of the brow with their fingers,[1] indicating that what they wish is the correction of brow ptosis (Flower's sign) (**Fig. 1**). Two of the characteristic age-related changes to the eyebrow are medial brow elevation and lateral brow ptosis.[2] These apparent changes may be a consequence of involution of the infraorbital soft tissues as much as actual positional changes of the brow itself as shown by Lambros. He examined the brow position of the averaged images of 169 young women (average age 24 years) against the averaged brow position for 145 older women (average age 76 years)[3] documenting the aforementioned findings. Consequently, multiple surgical techniques have focused on reversing these changes in an effort to achieve a more youthful and attractive appearance.

HISTORY

Brow lift surgery dates from 1919, when the anterior hairline brow lift was described.[4] This technique was followed by the coronal approach in 1962[5] and subsequently by the temporal scalp technique in 1973.[6] Later, in the early 1990s, the subgaleal endoscopic approach was introduced by Vasconez,[7] which remains popular to the present day. In addition, different planes of dissection and different brow lift approaches have also been proposed over the years including subperiosteal endoscopic, the subcutaneous hairline, and temporal approaches.[8–10]

Within a few years after the introduction of the endoscopic brow lift technique, surgeons began to question whether there was a correlation between the surgical outcomes and the esthetic ideals of the eyebrow height and shape.[11] The standard open and endoscopic brow lift operations oftentimes can result in unsatisfactory eyebrow height and shape. A frequent early finding with the endoscopic approach was excessive medial brow elevation and inadequate lateral brow correction. Suffice it to say, it is very easy

[a] Division of Plastic Surgery, University of Alabama at Birmingham, JNWB Suite 103, 500 22nd Street SouthBirmingham, AL 35233, USA; [b] Division of Plastic Surgery, University of Alabama at Birmingham, Grotting Plastic Surgery, One Inverness Center Parkway, Suite 100, Birmingham, AL 35242, USA
* Corresponding author.
E-mail address: jcgrotting@gmail.com

Clin Plastic Surg 49 (2022) 377–387
https://doi.org/10.1016/j.cps.2022.01.005
0094-1298/22/© 2022 Elsevier Inc. All rights reserved.

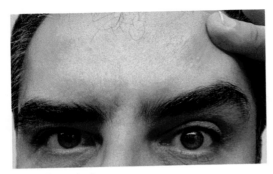

Fig. 1. Flower's sign.

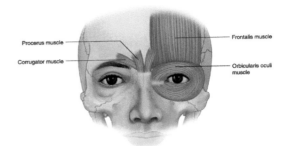

Fig. 2. Schematic view of the forehead anatomy. The key to forehead rejuvenation is releasing structures and repositioning them. (*From* Nierkrash CE. Chapter 8: Anatomy of the periorbital region. In: Fernieni, E. Applied Head and Neck Anatomy for the Facial Cosmetic Surgeon. 1st Ed. Springer; 2021:73-78.)

to over elevate the medial brow and is difficult to adequately elevate the lateral brow long term.

According to the ASPS National Plastic Surgery Procedural Statistics, the popularity of brow lift has decreased during the past decade. In 2000, it was the fifth most common cosmetic procedure performed in the United States with 120,971 cases. In 2019, a total of 89,246 brow lifts were performed, whereas in 2020, the number of reported brow lifts were 88,675, placing brow lift at the 10th most common esthetic operation performed that year in the United States. Overall, forehead lift surgery reduced by 27% between 2000 and 2020.

DEFINITIONS

The characteristics of the esthetically ideal brow are (1) the medial brow should be at or below the superior orbital rim; (2) the brow should peak lateral to the midpoint at roughly two-third of the length of the brow; and (3) the tail of the brow should be above the medial head of the brow in women. Therefore, when looking at models in various continents around the world from fashion magazines, one realizes that almost all of them have a very similar brow shape. The goal of brow lifting is to restore the brow to the aforementioned ideal anatomically ideal position. If the eyebrow shape is correctly achieved, it will be interpreted as beautiful even though it may be in a higher or lower location.

Brow lift is defined as a surgical procedure that reduces the rhytids that develop horizontally across the forehead, and the bridge of the nose (between the eyes), improves frown lines (the vertical creases that develop between the eyebrows), raises sagging brows that are hooding the upper eyelids, and places the eyebrows in an alert and youthful position.

BACKGROUND

The key to forehead rejuvenation is the adequate release with the restoration of the ideal brow position. (**Fig. 2**).When tailoring the brow position,

special attention should be paid to the shape more importantly than the height

Most patients benefit by lifting the tail of the brow and leaving the medial brow where it is, especially if it is already ideally positioned over the orbital rim. For this reason, temporal lift procedures have become much more popular in recent years. The coronal and endoscopic techniques release brow structures across the superior orbital rim and very often one sees unnatural elevation of the medial brow over time. Therefore, our preference is to reserve an endoscopic brow lift for those patients who would benefit by elevation of the medial brow. We abandoned coronal brow lifting decades ago.

In an effort to find a reliable way to elevate the temporal brow with predictability and durability, we have adapted Fausto Viterbo's gliding brow lift (GBL) in most of our patients who require brow shaping or brow lifting laterally. The technique continues to evolve but it is remarkable how much control one has over brow shape as well as elevation of the soft tissues of the temporal region lateral to the orbit. In fact, one can even elevate the lateral canthus using this technique.

DISCUSSION

The eyebrow is a surface structure on a gliding subcutaneous plane (Video 1).

The subcutaneous technique has been advocated by different authors because of the reduced need for specialized instruments or osseous fixation. The subcutaneous plane is associated with decreased complications more commonly seen in other techniques such as frontal branch injury, and raising of the hairline and edema. Other advantages described in the subcutaneous dissection are better control and lower tension of brow suspension, quicker recovery with predictable preservation of results. The temporal subcutaneous approach has also produced consistent results with low risks.[12]

Risks and complications may occur after any surgery even if well executed. The most common observed complication after a facelift is hematoma,[13] and this usually happens within the first 48 postoperative hours.[14] As a means of preventing this known complication, the concept of the auersvald hemostatic net was applied to neck lift and facelift,[15] which was adapted from other techniques, such as quilting sutures. The quilting sutures technique was first reported in the ophthalmic British literature in 1979 for periorbital skin graft fixation.[16] The use of quilting sutures is now widely used in abdominoplasty and the transcutaneous hemostatic net has been adapted widely for face and neck lifting as previously mentioned. After our very positive experience using the hemostatic net for preventing hematoma and skin repositioning in facelifting, we began to use the technique for subcutaneous brow lifting according to the technique introduced by Fausto Viterbo.[17]

Subcutaneous undermining is not a new technique, but the GBL differs from other temporal subcutaneous techniques by undermining immediately above the frontalis and galea in a blind manner using blunt dissectors to separate and subsequently hold the brow in the desired shape and keep it there with the hemostatic net. The net will elevate the lower portion of the brow and at the same time accommodate the skin excess on the upper portion of the brow. The transcutaneous sutures are removed 2 to 3 days after surgery (**Fig. 3**).

This technique provides the advantage of having almost no scars and 2 different effects, skin elongation followed by skin shrinkage. Other benefits of this procedure are the ability to elevate the brow without increasing the forehead height, it also provides a Botox-like effect by separating the subcutaneous layer from the corrugators with minimal risk of hematoma. Potential complications of GBL like all brow lifting procedures are brow asymmetry, skin necrosis, relapse and exacerbation of preexisting ptosis.

Dr Grotting's Experience

The senior author (JCG) has a 26-year experience performing the endoscopic brow lift using a variety of modifications (**Fig. 4**).

Looking at long-term results, the technique seems to work well for the elevation of the medial brow. We now reserve the endoscopic brow lift for very specific patients—that is, those who require elevation of the medial brow or patients who have very heavy, hyperdynamic glabellar musculature (**Fig. 5**).

Unsatisfactory long-term results have been observed with the endoscopic brow lift technique, leading to elevation of the medial brow and poor durability of elevation of the lateral brow (**Figs. 6 and 7**).

In patients who do not require elevation of the medial brow, we now favor the use of Fausto Viterbo's GBL. We have been using the GBL for the past 2.5 years with good outcomes.

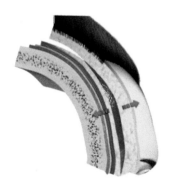
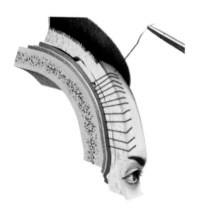

Fig. 3. Plane of dissection and application of hemostatic net. Figure on the left shows a cross-section of the subcutaneous tissues that are elevated. On the right, the galea and frontalis muscles are fixated using the hemostatic net suture technique. (*Adapted from* Viterbo F, Auersvald A, O'Daniel TG. Gliding Brow Lift (GBL): A New Concept. Aesthetic Plast Surg. 2019 Dec;43(6):1536–1546.)

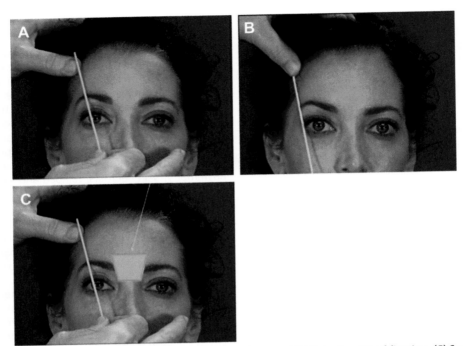

Fig. 4. Principles of brow fixation using the endoscopic technique. (*A*) Highest point of fixation. (*B*) Second point of fixation, the lateral tail. (*C*) Green area represents the region where the periosteum should be maintained, and muscles disinserted.

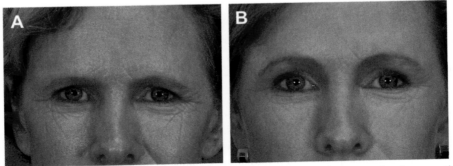

Fig. 5. 38-year-old female with a history of significant sun exposure. Patient has a very low brow position. She is an excellent candidate for using the endoscopic technique to elevate the medial and lateral brow. (*A*) Preoperative appearance. (*B*) Postoperative appearance after 1 year.

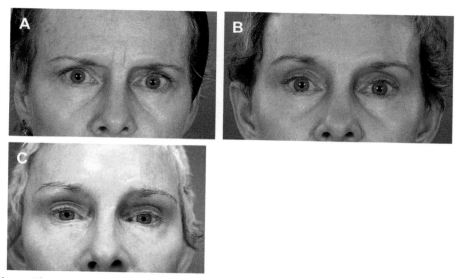

Fig. 6. Patient with very low medial brow position and heavy corrugator and procerus musculature. (*A*) Preoperative photograph. (*B*) Early postoperative appearance after endoscopic brow lift and blepharoplasty. (*C*) Patient's appearance 12 years after surgery, showing medial brow elevation and poor lateral lift.

Other application of the GBL technique is for the treatment of temporal bunching following facelifting.

Operative Technique

Access incisions are planned according to the height of the hairline and the position of the sideburn.

In many patients, the entire undermining can be accomplished through a single access site behind the hairline superiorly. In other patients, a second access site is helpful in the sideburn area. We outline the area to be dissected *with* a marking pen (**Fig. 8**).

The procedure can be performed under local anesthesia or general, especially if other procedures are being performed in the face. Using an 18-gauge needle, approximately 60 cc of tumescent solution is infiltrated in the subcutaneous plane on each side of thee forehead. It is imperative that the subcutaneous plane be maximally distended with the tumescent fluid. This ensures that one does not inadvertently pass through the galea or frontalis muscle during the blunt blind dissection. We usually do the right side first and do not tumesce the left side until we are ready to begin the undermining (Video 2).

A 3-mm stab incision is made in the hairline on each side and widened with a hemostat. We

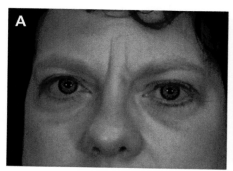
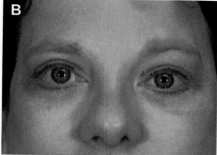

Fig. 7. Patient status post endoscopic brow lift with a modest elevation of the lateral brow but improvement of the medial proposition. (*A*) Preoperative photograph of a patient with a low medial brow. (*B*) Medial brow has been raised after modification of corrugator and procerus.

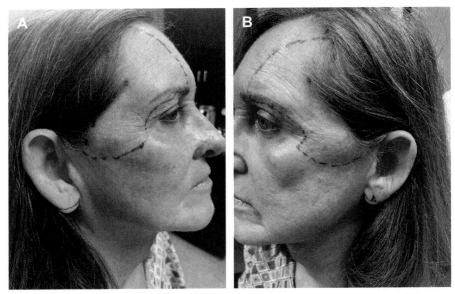

Fig. 8. Preoperative markings for gliding brow lift technique. (*A*) Right lateral view. (*B*) Left lateral view.

proceed to undermining with the Viterbo dissectors. First, the straight dissector is inserted to dissect inferiorly toward and just below the lateral brow. Then, the curved dissector is used to free up any remaining subcutaneous soft tissue attachments in the transverse direction, and finally, the right-angle "hockey stick" dissector is used (**Fig. 9**).

We generally work from medial to lateral so that the temporal line of fusion can be taken down and the lateral orbital tissues down to the zygomatic arch. In fact, dissection can proceed inferior to the arch if one desires to elevate the malar region as well.

There is often bleeding associated with this blunt dissection and all the blood is simply expressed from the access site before placing the net.

Two skin hooks are used to place the brow exactly in the shape and position desired. The first 2 sutures placed are within the eyebrow itself. We then place a 4-0 Prolene suture through the brow extending down to the deeper soft tissues at the superior orbital rim close to the periosteum. These 2 individual sutures stay for 5 days.

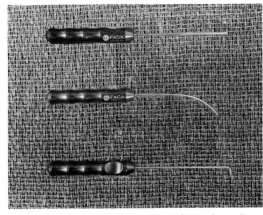

Fig. 9. The three different types of Viterbo's dissectors: straight, curve, and right angle. (*From* Faga Medical.)

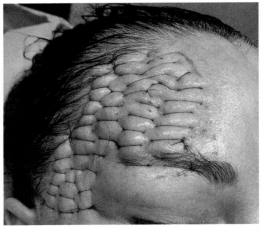

Fig. 10. Patient with Auersvald hemostatic net holding the tissues in place during gliding brow lift surgery.

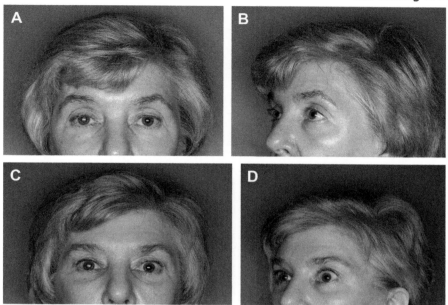

Fig. 11. 78-year-old patient status after facelift, gliding brow lift, and autologous fat grafting. She improved her brow shape by elevation of the temporal brow without elevation of the medial brow. (*A, B*) Preoperative appearance. (*C, D*) Patient's appearance at 3 months follow-up.

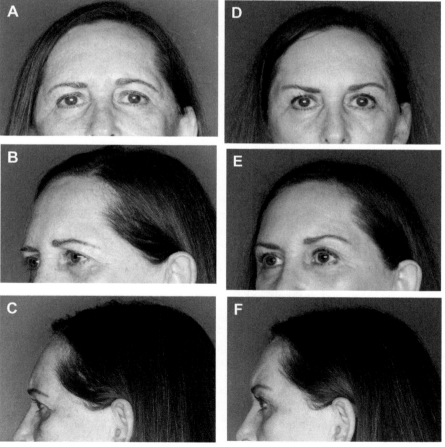

Fig. 12. Improvement in brow shape in the temporal area, using the gliding brow lift technique. (*A, B, C*) Preoperative appearance. (*D, E, F*) Appearance at 3 months postoperatively.

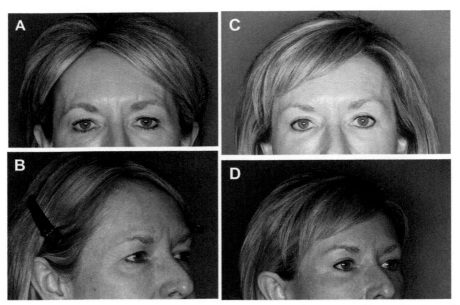

Fig. 13. Patient who underwent facelift, gliding brow lift, deep neck lift, upper and lower blepharoplasty. (*A, B*) Preoperative appearance. (*C, D*) Postoperative appearance at 1 year follow-up.

We then place the running 5-0 Prolene net sutures starting in the temporal region and extending superiorly to the hairline. The sutures are placed in rows approximately 2 cm apart avoiding significant tension. Care is taken to angle the needle parallel to the course of the frontal branch to minimize the possibility of trapping or injuring the nerve. We have had no permanent frontal branch injuries. The suture is on a 25-mm sharp taper point needle to make certain that the underlying galea and frontalis muscle are incorporated into the running suture. The sutures are placed in rows until the entire area that was undermined is fixed in position. In this manner, the dead space is closed, encouraging adhesion and obliteration of the created space. Usually, about 4 to 5 rows of sutures are placed (**Fig. 10**). If bunching occurs at the hairline, a second pocket below the galea under the hair-bearing scalp can be created using the technique of Ozan Sozer.[18] Using a suture like a Gigli saw, the subcutaneous space can be communicated with the subgaleal space lateral to the hairline in order to reposition the hair-bearing scalp and hold it in position but we have found this to be rarely necessary. It is essential that the assistant hold the skin hooks with the precise amount of tension to create symmetry on both sides. The scalp is retracted strongly superiorly,

and a little overcorrection is desirable as there is always some dissent when the patient goes from supine to upright. If modification of the corrugator and procerus muscles is indicated, this can be performed directly via the transblepharoplasty approach, but in most cases, patients are treated with neurotoxin.

Once the right side is completed, attention is turned to the left side and an identical mirror image correction is performed. The stab incisions are closed with a simple nylon suture. Usually, a light dressing is helpful simply to help the patient and family tolerate the sutures without having to see them. The net sutures are removed at 2 days by cutting the knots out and then simply cutting each suture in the middle and taking out each of the small remaining bites. The 2 interrupted sutures in the brow are left for 5 days. We have had no issues with visible scarring from the sutures or hyperpigmentation.

GBL can be performed as a primary procedure (**Figs. 11** and **12**) or in conjunction with other operations that are being primarily (**Figs. 13** and **14**).

As mentioned earlier, the GBL procedure can also be carried out as a secondary operation to correct temporal bunching (Video 3).

We have seen a few cases of failure of GBL in our case series, in those cases, direct brow lift was used to correct failure (**Fig. 15**).

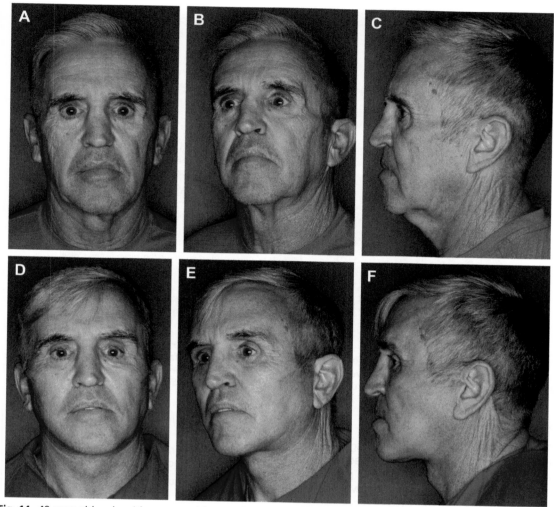

Fig. 14. 49-year-old male with a remote history of facial trauma (bilateral LeFort I, II, and III). He underwent face-lift, deep cervicoplasty, gliding brow lift, and autologous fat grafting in the periorbital region. (*A, B, C*) Preoperative photographs. (*D, E, F*) Postoperative photographs demonstrating improvement of brow shape in addition to correction of lagophthalmos.

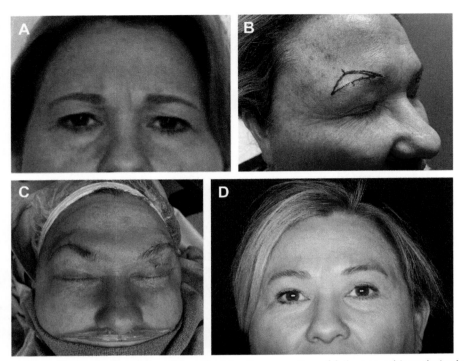

Fig. 15. Direct brow lift was performed on this patient for the correction of failure to achieve desired outcomes with the GBL technique. (*A*) Preoperative appearance after GBL. (*B*) Direct brow lift preoperative markings. (*C*) Intraoperative photographs after completion of suturing. (*D*) Postoperative appearance.

SUMMARY

The brow undergoes noticeable changes secondary to aging. To the standard observer, brow shape is more important than brow position, so most women benefit by selective elevation of the tail of the brow. As the medial brow tends to elevate with age, surgeons should be careful to use techniques that do not lift the medial brow above the supraorbital rim, which may happen with the endoscopic or coronal technique.

Good and reproducible results are achievable working in the subcutaneous plane with solid, temporary fixation (Viterbo's GBL technique).

There is no generalizable brow lift; therefore, techniques used must be suited to the esthetic goals of the patient and comfort level of the surgeon.

CLINICS CARE POINTS

- Can be performed under local anesthesia comfortably
- Minimal incision and subcutaneous brow lift techniques are not new—but using the Auersvald hemostatic net to hold the

elevated structures in place is a novel advancement
- The gliding brow lift can be used to address temporal bunching after facelift
- Glabellar musculature can be treated through a transblepharoplasty approach or with neurotoxins
- Unsatisfactory results are not the fault of the technique necessarily but usually due to poor patient selection or how the technique is applied

DISCLOSURE

Side relationships: Founder CosmetAssure, which is owned by Aesthetic Surgeons Financial Group—Shareholder. Affiliations: ASAPS, CME editor, Aesthetic Surgery Journal Editorial Board, The Breast Journal, Brijjit LLC, Engage Media, Vita Group LLC; Compensation: Aesthetic Surgeons Financial Group officer; Other: Thieme Publishing, Elsevier.

SUPPLEMENTARY DATA

Supplementary data related to this article can be found online at https://doi.org/10.1016/j.cps.2022.01.005.

REFERENCES

1. Marten TJ, Elyassnia D. In: Farhadieh RD, Bulstrode NW, Mehrara BJ, et al, editors. "Forehead lift". plastic surgery - principles and practice. Elsevier; 2022. p. 973–1007.
2. Matros E, Garcia JA, Yaremchuk MJ. Changes in eyebrow position and shape with aging. Plast Reconstr Surg 2009;124(4):1296–301.
3. Lambros V. Facial aging: a 54-year, three-dimensional population study. Plast Reconstr Surg 2020;145(4):921–8.
4. Passot R. La chururgie essthetique des rides du visage. Press Med 1919;27:258.
5. Gonzales-Ulloah M. Facial wrinkles: integral elimination. Plast Reconstr Surg 1962;29:658–73.
6. Gleason MC. Brow lifting through a temporal scalp approach. Plast Reconstr Surg 1973;52(2):141–4.
7. Vasconez L, Core G, Gamboa-Bobadilla M, et al. Endoscopic techniques in coronal brow lifting. Plast Reconstr Surg 1994;94(6):788–93.
8. Knize DM. Reassessment of the coronal incision and subgaleal dissection for foreheadplasty. Plast Reconstr Surg 1998;102(2):478–89 [discussion: 490-2].
9. Tessier P. Le lifting facial sous-périosté [Subperiosteal face-lift]. Ann Chir Plast Esthet 1989;34(3):193–7.
10. Guyuron B, Davies B. Subcutaneous anterior hairline forehead rhytidectomy. Aesthetic Plast Surg 1988; 12:77.
11. Freund RM, Nolan WB 3rd. Correlation between brow lift outcomes and aesthetic ideals for eyebrow height and shape in females. Plast Reconstr Surg 1996;97(7):1343–8.
12. Savetsky IL, Matarasso A. Lateral temporal subcutaneous brow lift: clinical experience and systematic review of the literature. Plast Reconstr Surg Glob Open 2020;8(4):e2764.
13. Baker TJ, Gordon HL. Complications of rhytidectomy. Plast Reconstr Surg 1967;40:31.
14. Rees TD, Barone CM, Valauri FA, et al. Hematomas requiring surgical evacuation following face lift surgery. Plast Reconstr Surg 1994;93(6):1185–90.
15. Auersvald A, Auersvald LA. Hemostatic net in rhytidoplasty: an efficient and safe method for preventing hematoma in 405 consecutive patients. Aesthetic Plast Surg 2014;38(1):1–9.
16. Mehta HK. A new method of full thickness skin graft fixation. Br J Ophthalmol 1979;63(2):125–8.
17. Viterbo F, Auersvald A, O'Daniel TG. Gliding brow lift (GBL): a new concept. Aesthet Plast Surg 2019; 43(6):1536–46.
18. Erol OO, Sozer SO, Velidedeoglu HV. Brow suspension, a minimally invasive technique in facial rejuvenation. Plast Reconstr Surg 2002;109(7):2521–32 [discussion: 2533].

Creating Harmonious Arcs
The Importance of Brow Shape in Determining Upper Lid Aesthetics

Mohammed S. Alghoul, MD, FACS[a,b,]*, Elbert E. Vaca, MD[c]

KEYWORDS

• Brow shaping • Upper blepharoplasty • Brow aesthetics • Periorbital

KEY POINTS

- The three-dimensional surface topography of the brow–upper eyelid aesthetic unit consists of harmonious arcs and spaces, which determine the perception of attractiveness of the periorbital area.
- The ideal brow shape, which has a direct impact on the upper lid fold shape and height, starts low medially and ascends in a gentle curve peaking at the level of the lateral canthus. The upper lid fold starts short and flat medially and transitions into youthful convexity laterally.
- Shaping the upper lid fold is critical for shaping the temporal brow.

INTRODUCTION

There are several described approaches for brow and upper eyelid rejuvenation.[1–21] Although the technique used varies based on the individual surgeon's training and experience, it is the aesthetic judgment that is most important to obtain consistent results. In our opinion, a greater emphasis needs to be placed on the preoperative aesthetic assessment; this analysis serves as the foundation to individually titrate the operation to aesthetically shape the brow. Furthermore, the brow is only one component of the upper periorbital unit. The upper lid, specifically the upper lid fold volume and topographic contour, the curvature of the upper eyelid crease and brow, and the presence of ptosis must be critically analyzed.[1–3,22] To that end, this article reviews upper periorbital aesthetics, anatomy, and the authors' preferred approach to shape the brow and upper periorbital area, when indicated, to optimize aesthetic outcomes.

IDEAL UPPER PERIORBITAL AESTHETICS

Everything should be made as simple as possible, but not simpler

—Albert Einstein

Based on periorbital aesthetic analysis studies performed by our group,[1,22] we have demonstrated that patients can present with varying combinations of upper lid aging aberrations. As a result, execution of a "one size fits all" approach to upper periorbital surgery risks a poor aesthetic outcome.[1,2] A higher-level understanding of upper periorbital aesthetics is essential for a more thoughtful preoperative analysis as a means to tailor the appropriate surgical approach to the patient's individual anatomy and aesthetic concerns.

UPPER LID ARCS AND SPACES

The upper periorbital area is thought of as a series of three interrelated arcs including the upper lid

a Private Practice, Abdali Hospital, 12th floor, Al-Istethmar Street, Abdali Boulevar, Amman 11190, Jordan;
b Division of Plastic & Reconstructive Surgery, Northwestern Feinberg School of Medicine, 675 N Street Clair, Galter 250, IL 60611, Chicago; c Private Practice, 660 Glades Road, Suite 210, Boca Raton, FL 33431, USA
* Corresponding author. Private Practice, Abdali Hospital, 12th floor, Al-Istethmar Street, Abdali Boulevar, Amman 11190, Jordan.
E-mail address: Mo.Alghoul@gmail.com

Clin Plastic Surg 49 (2022) 389–397
https://doi.org/10.1016/j.cps.2022.01.006
0094-1298/22/© 2022 Elsevier Inc. All rights reserved.

margin, the upper lid crease, and the brow; the pretarsal space and upper lid fold are the intervening spaces between these arcs, respectively (**Fig. 1**).[1,3,22] The upper lid margin should cover the upper scleral limbus and lie approximately 4 mm above the center of the pupil (ie, marginal reflex distance 1 [MRD1]). MRD1 discrepancies greater than 0.5 mm and/or MRD1 less than or equal to 3 mm are perceived as upper lid ptosis and can convey a tired, aged appearance.

The curvatures of the upper lid arcs are critical for the perceived youth and attractiveness of the periorbital area. These curvatures should form smooth arcs, with the exception of a slightly more pronounced inflection point of the brow arc corresponding to the brow peak. In females, the arc peaks should progressively lateralize, with the lid margin peak located approximately 1 mm lateral to the midpupil, the lid crease peak approximately 2 mm lateral to the midpupil, and the brow peak located at approximately the level of the lateral canthus (see **Fig. 1**).[22] The aged and less attractive eye is characterized by aberrations of these curvatures including an increased prevalence of upper lid ptosis, medialization and a more pronounced inflection point (ie, A-frame deformity) of the upper lid crease peak,[1,2,22] and lateral brow ptosis, which results in medialization of the brow peak (**Fig. 2**A).

An attractive smooth curvature of the upper lid crease consequently results in an even height (from nasal to lateral) of the youthful appearing pretarsal space (**Fig. 2**B). The attractive upper lid fold, however, gradually increases in height laterally with its maximum height located at approximately the lateral canthus corresponding to the apex of the ideal brow arc. Although the amount of pretarsal show can vary significantly among attractive subjects, it is a consistent feature of attractive female eyes that the upper lid fold to pretarsal show ratios should increase from the medial to lateral aspects of the lid. This is caused by the lateral brow peak with attractive downward angulation of the medial brow (**Fig. 3**B). In the aged and less attractive eye, a medialized and more pronounced acuity of the upper lid crease peak results in loss of the homogeneous height of the pretarsal space (see **Fig. 2**A; **Fig. 3**A). This is further exacerbated by lateral brow ptosis resulting in loss of lateral pretarsal show. Similarly, lateral brow descent results in loss of the vertical height of the lateral upper lid fold and medialization of the brow peak, resulting in a loss of youthful upper lid fold to pretarsal show ratios (see **Fig. 2**A).

The youthful surface topography of the upper lid fold also varies from nasal to lateral, with a flat contour medial to the pupil and a gradual increase in convexity of the lateral upper lid fold and brow (see **Fig. 3**B). With aging, herniation or bulges of the nasal orbital fat and volumetric deflation of the lateral upper lid fold fat (ie, retro-orbicularis oculi fat [ROOF]) results in a disruption of the youthful upper lid fold contour. It is critical to note that upper eyelid aging can occur in different patterns caused by varying degrees of dermatochalasis, upper lid ptosis, the patient's globe vector, brow position, and localized upper lid fold volumetric deficiency or excess. Excess visible pretarsal show can result in a tired and gaunt appearance and occur because of a combination upper lid ptosis, periorbital volume loss, and compensatory brow strain caused by ptosis. Meanwhile, other patients can demonstrate "heavy" appearing upper lids caused by a potential combination of severe dermatochalasis and brow ptosis that can result in opacification of their pretarsal space. A prior study by our group demonstrated that patients with greater than 4 mm of pretarsal show had worse aesthetic ratings; traditional excisional blepharoplasty in patients with preexisting pretarsal show excess is a high risk of a poor cosmetic outcome. Therefore, recognition of the aging pattern is critical to tailor the operation to optimize results.[1]

BROW SHAPE

Turning our attention back to the brow, the brow is best thought of as the "frame" of the eye and is a critical reference point by which the attractiveness of the eye itself is judged. In females, the lateral apex and gentle medial downward angulation is a key attractive feature. In a retrospective analysis of 316 patients who underwent upper blepharoplasty, 62% of patients presented with unfavorable brow aesthetics (defined as the inferior brow margin at the lateral orbital rim being lower than the brow at the medial canthus; see **Fig. 2**A); these patients had significantly worse preoperative and postoperative aesthetic scores. Importantly, patients with unfavorable brows who underwent brow lift had significantly better postoperative scores than those who did not. In addition, brow lifting resulted in lateralization of the apex of the brow arc.[1] Hence, in the appropriate patient, brow lifting is a critical element to optimize the aesthetic outcome (see **Fig. 2**B).

It is critical to understand the difference between brow shape, brow position, and the different variables that influence each of them. Although a brow position located above the supraorbital rim is considered more aesthetic in females, the brow must also follow a certain curvature and angulation to have a favorable shape, as detailed

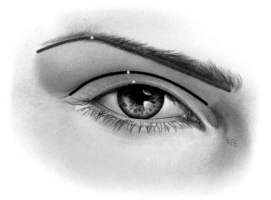

Fig. 1. The three upper lid arcs are the lid margin (*red*), the upper lid crease (*black*), and the inferior margin of the brow (*blue*). There is a progressive lateralization of the peaks of the lid margin, crease, and brow arcs, respectively, in the attractive eye. The pretarsal space has a uniform height from medial to lateral, whereas the upper lid fold height increases from medial to lateral peaking at the lateral canthus with the brow peak. The surface topography of the upper lid fold changes from flat medially to more convex laterally. (*Courtesy of* Levent Efe, Brunswick, AU.)

previously. Any deviation from the attractive shape should raise the question of an underlying eyelid pathology. For example, patients with upper lid ptosis often present with a high brow that has an abnormal curvature where the peak is medialized. This is caused by a compensatory frontalis strain favoring the medial brow to elevate the upper lid, therefore altering the shape and creating brow

position asymmetry. Similarly, asymmetry in hemifacial orbital bony anatomy can result in unilateral brow ptosis on the side with orbital rim recession.

SURGICAL UPPER PERIORBITAL ANATOMY
Tissue Layers

Temple and forehead anatomy is complex with varying terminology, nerves that change planes along their course, and areas of adhesion to the underlying periosteum.[23–25] Although several of these details are outside the scope of this article, from an aesthetic surgical perspective, the forehead and temple are comprised of distinct tissue layers including: (1) skin, (2) subcutaneous fat, (3) superficial fascia (superficial temporal fascia, which is continuous with the frontalis muscle medially), (4) subfascial fat (subgaleal/subfrontalis fat in the forehead; superficial temporal fat pad lateral to the superior temporal line of fusion), (5) innominate fascia (also termed "loose areolar tissue," which is continuous with the parotidmasseteric fascia), (6) deep temporal fascia (ie, overlying fascia of the temporalis muscle; this layer fuses with the periosteum at the superior temporal line of fusion), and (7) periosteum.

Retaining Ligaments of the Temporal and Periorbital Area

The superior temporal septum, or line of fusion, is a circumlinear area of adhesion to the underlying periosteum located at the cephalad periosteal insertion of the temporalis muscle.[25] Medially, approaching the superolateral orbital rim, this area of adhesion to the periosteum broadens and

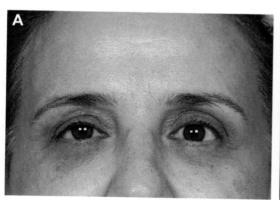
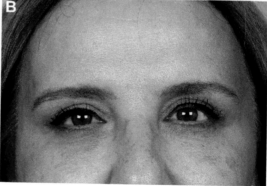

Fig. 2. Preoperative and 6-month postoperative results in a 55-year-old female patient who underwent simultaneous temporal subcutaneous, upper blepharoplasty with fat shifting and muscle contouring, and ptosis repair with Muller muscle resection. (*A*) Preoperative photograph showing unfavorable brow shape with medialization of the peak of the brow caused by frontalis strain elevating the ptotic lid margin, asymmetric and nonuniform height of the pretarsal space with decreased upper lid fold. Pretarsal space medially and A-frame deformity and decreased MRD1 distance mainly on the right side. (*B*) Postoperative photograph showing more harmonious arcs and uniform spaces with more attractive proportions.

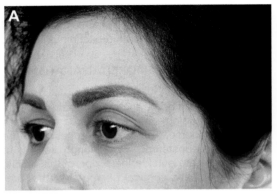
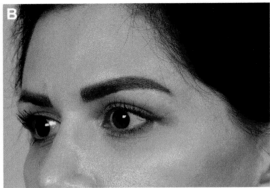

Fig. 3. Preoperative and 8-month postoperative results in a 48-year-old female patient, oblique view, who underwent temporal brow lift, upper blepharoplasty with fat grafting and muscle contouring, and ptosis repair with Muller muscle resection. (*A*) Preoperative photograph showing increased pretarsal show and ill-defined upper lid fold. (*B*) Postoperative photograph showing a distinct pretarsal space with decreased and more uniform height, and a more defined upper lid fold with a flat contour medially transitioning to youthful convexity laterally.

becomes more robust. This area is called the temporal ligamentous adhesion and supraorbital ligamentous adhesion further medially, as described by Moss and colleagues.[25,26]

The orbicularis retaining ligament (ORL) is an osteocutaneous ligament that originates from the orbital rim periosteum just outside the origin of the orbital septum. The ORL courses through the orbicularis oculi muscle and then has fibers that attach to the overlying dermis, forming a septal attachment to the underlying periosteum in a C-shaped configuration beginning at approximately the medial scleral limbus.[27–32] Laterally, the ORL terminates and fuses with the orbital septum as a fibrous thickening called the lateral orbital thickening, also known as the superficial lateral canthal tendon.[28,33]

Neurovascular Structures

The supraorbital nerve emerges from the supraorbital notch (or foramen) approximately 1 cm lateral to the medial brow margin and divides into superficial and deep nerve branches. The superficial nerve branch courses in a mostly superior vector and divides into several branches that enter the subcutaneous plane approximately 2.6 cm above the superior orbital rim. Along their course, these branches either pierce the corrugator supercilii muscle or pierce the frontalis muscle just cephalad to the corrugator. The deep branch courses superolaterally deep to the corrugator and frontalis muscles and lies medial to the superior temporal line of fusion.[34,35] The frontal branch of the facial nerve first courses deep to the innominate fascia and then transitions to the deep surface of the superficial temporal fascia 1.5 to 3.0 cm above the

zygomatic arch, with its branches innervating the frontalis muscle along its deep surface.[24,36]

The superficial temporal, supratrochlear, and supraorbital vessels exhibit extensive and variable anastomoses in the frontalis muscle and superficial temporal fascia. The sentinel vein drains into the middle temporal vein and pierces from the superficial temporal fascia though the deep temporal fascia approximately 1 to 1.5 cm lateral to the zygomaticofrontal suture. Of note, the sentinel vein is located approximately 2 to 9 mm caudal to the course of the frontal branch of the facial nerve.[37] The zygomaticofrontal nerve (which originates from the maxillary division of the trigeminal nerve) pierces the deep temporal fascia to innervate the overlying temple skin approximately 1 cm lateral to the sentinel vein.[23,37]

Upper Lid Fold

The lateral upper lid fold volume is formed by the orbicularis oculi muscle, the central orbital fat pad, and the ROOF. These structures contribute the youthful and attractive convexity of this area. This area blends with the temporal fat posteriorly and tapers off inferiorly over the area of the lateral orbital thickening at the lateral canthus. The ROOF is a well-defined and enclosed fat compartment that measures approximately 1 cm × 4 cm.[38] Inferiorly, the ROOF is bounded by the robust ORL, which arises from the arcus marginalis. Superiorly, the ROOF is bounded by an area of fusion of orbicularis oculi muscle fibers to the frontalis muscle. Medially, the ROOF compartment gradually tapers, and the medial upper lid fold volume is formed mainly by the nasal orbital fat pad and preseptal fat (**Fig. 4**).[2,38]

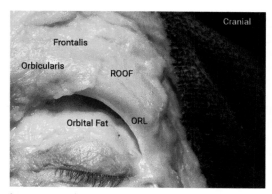

Fig. 4. Fresh frozen cadaver head, 77-year-old man, showing the brow anatomy.

Aesthetic Interdependence of the Upper Lid Fold and Brow

The upper eyelid and brow should be viewed as a single aesthetic unit. Correcting the brow shape and position has a direct impact on the shape and vertical height of the upper lid fold. Because these two structures are continuous, it is critical that their surface contour be addressed after setting the final brow position to achieve the best cosmetic outcomes. Together they form the superior limb of the C-angle.[38] Upper lid fold aging changes negatively impact the shape of the lid crease arc where both dermatochalasis and medial hollowing result in lid crease peak medialization. Medialization and increased acuity of the upper lid crease is further exacerbated by bulging of nasal orbital fat, contributing to what is known as the "A-frame" deformity. Lateral hooding, however, is a direct result of lateral brow descent, dermatochalasis, and potentially compounded by ROOF compartment volumetric atrophy. This can result in an increased acuity (or closure) of the lateral orbital area (C-angle) and loss of the convex contour of the lateral brow and upper lid fold. This may require a potential combination of a temporal brow lift, manipulation of deep structures to restore a more youthful contour (ie, orbital fat shifting or orbicularis muscle manipulation), and potential volumization via fat grafting.

Surgical Techniques to Shape the Upper Lid Fold

Brow lifting and shaping is an integral component of upper eyelid rejuvenation and should be combined with upper blepharoplasty, ptosis repair, and fat grafting, as needed, to create attractive harmonious arcs. Over the past 3 years, the authors started combining these approaches, oftentimes performing them in the same setting, to achieve the desired attractive topographic proportions and contours. Temporal brow lift is a powerful technique that expands the vertical height of the lateral upper lid fold, lateralizes the brow peak, and addresses lateral hooding. The latter is a frequently encountered sign of periorbital aging and is otherwise addressed with extended upper blepharoplasty in cases where the patient already has adequate upper lid fold height or has a brow tattoo with an artificially elevated tail. The procedure is performed in the subcutaneous or deep planes (discussed elsewhere in this issue). It is critical to note that brow lifting must be considered more than just a "lifting" procedure. It is more properly thought as a brow arc "shaping" operation. As such, the brow lift incision is centered about the intended brow apex (approximately at the level of the lateral canthus as a means to youthfully lateralize the brow peak) and extended medially and laterally to this point, as needed. The maximum vector of pull is exerted at the intended brow apex. Following this, the remainder of the brow is lifted and contoured incrementally to achieve a pleasing curvature. Of note, the incision often needs to be extended further laterally in patients with a greater degree of lateral hooding. In patients with a high temporal hairline, a subcutaneous pretrichial approach is recommended; meanwhile, in patients with a low temporal hairline, the lateral aspect of the incision is transitioned to a posthairline incision and dissection is performed in a subcutaneous versus deep plane. Direct temporal brow lift is another important technique in male patients who often have heavy, ptotic, and unstable temporal brows. When executed carefully, the scar is hidden in the hairline, usually heals well, and is inconspicuous compared with the more visible extended version over the medial brow.

Although temporal brow lift lays the foundation for establishing lateral upper lid fold height and shape, ptosis repair similarly lays the foundation for tensioning the lid margin and shortening the pretarsal space. In patients with good levator function who show good response to phenylephrine eye drops, Muller muscle resection is an excellent technique that predictably elevates the upper lid margin while minimizing contour irregularities. If blepharoptosis is accompanied by medial elevation of the brow, it is the authors' opinion that a temporal brow lift or brow shaping procedure should be considered at the same time of ptosis correction because this brow peak medialization does not always self-correct after ptosis repair. Several surgical maneuvers are applied to shape the brow–eyelid fold subunit to enhance a youthful convexity laterally while keeping a short flat segment medially.

Orbital Fat Manipulation and Fat Shifting

Fat shifting uses the existing configuration of the orbital fat to improve the surface topography of the upper lid fold and brow. In principle, fat shifting is a medial to lateral shift of the orbital fat compartments to transfer the upper lid fold volume from where it is less desired medially to where it is more desired laterally. After the skin is excised, a narrow strip of orbicularis is excised along the entire width of the incision, widening laterally. Suborbicularis oculi muscle dissection is performed until the superolateral orbital rim is reached and the ORL is encountered. The ORL is a strong septum that forms the inferior boundary of the ROOF compartment. The ORL is divided, and the ROOF is exposed. Following that the orbital septum is opened and the preaponeurotic, central fat pad, and the nasal fat pads are mobilized. The central fat pad has an orange-yellow color and is easier to mobilize where it reaches the ROOF easily. It is then laid over the ROOF compartment and the degree of augmentation, and therefore the amount to be transferred is determined. The orbital fat is transferred as a flap and is kept attached to its pedicle. Fixation is performed using interrupted sutures making sure not to cover the arcus marginalis at the vertical level of the lateral canthus because this acts as a fixation point to the muscle later. Shifting the central fat pad or part of it laterally typically creates a volume void centrally. The nasal fat pad is mobilized next.[39] Using a small retractor medially and retropulsion helps identify its location. It is typically more fibrous, has a pale-yellow color, and is located more medial and inferior. Extensive mobilization of the nasal fat pad is required for it to be transferred laterally to augment the central fold (**Fig. 5**). Failure to do so can result in retraction of the fat pad back to its original location. Fixation is performed next to the arcus marginalis and to the central fat pad. Further tensioning with sutures is carried on until the desired contour is reached. Fat shifting is performed to sculpt the entire fold or is targeted to improve localized volume deficiency in the fold as in the A-frame deformity. Another alternative is to simply excise the fat responsible for the medial bulge, which is typically comprised of the nasal fat pad and medial portion of the central fat pad; leave the remaining central fat pad and septum undisturbed; and to fat graft the ROOF and sulcus to achieve similar contour. In some patients with heavy upper lid folds, fat excision is performed of the nasal and central fat pads and muscle contouring is used primarily to create the differential surface contour from medial to lateral.

Orbicularis Contouring

Orbicularis oculi muscle excision has been one of the controversial steps in upper blepharoplasty over the past few decades with its value being questioned by many. In the authors' opinion, it is not simply a matter of excision but contouring that gives the orbicularis an important role in upper lid fold shaping. Not every patient requires muscle excision; fat manipulation is performed by incising the muscle creating localized windows. Younger patients usually do not require muscle excision and the muscle is preserved to maintain a youthful volume. Two particularly useful maneuvers that enhance upper lid fold–brow shape are muscle tightening medially and inversion laterally. After a strip of muscle is removed or simple muscle incision, and following fat manipulation, muscle tightening is performed on the medial most extent of the incision. The muscle edges are imbricated, which brings the cut skin edges in direct contact and creates an immediate flattening effect on the medial fold. Over the midpupillary line, the muscle is either left undisturbed, plicated, approximated end to end if an incision or excision are performed, or sutured to the levator aponeurosis in cases of concomitant ptosis repair. At the level of the lateral canthus, the arcus marginalis is exposed by dissecting in a suborbicularis plane toward the superolateral orbital rim. The superior and inferior edges of the orbicularis oculi are sewn to the arcus marginalis in a buried fashion causing a tucking or inversion effect of the fold and therefore enhancing the convexity of the upper lid fold laterally (**Fig. 6**). This technique was originally described in similar form by Zarem and colleagues[40] as a brow fixation maneuver. If fat shifting is performed at the same time, care is taken not to compromise the blood supply of the transferred fat flap. It is important not to extend this maneuver beyond the lateral canthus because this may create an abnormal fold shape in that area. Alternatively, the orbicularis edges are approximated to the arcus marginalis starting at the medial extent of the incision, creating tightening, and flattening medially, and then continued in a running fashion until the lateral canthus is reached. Lateral to the lateral canthus, simple approximation of the muscle edges in performed.

Fat Grafting

Fat grafting is a great tool to volumize and contour the upper lid–brow complex.[41] Because the ROOF is a well-contained compartment with well-defined boundaries, it is easily fat grafted and reliably augmented to create the desired convexity of the lateral fold. If this is planned, the ROOF

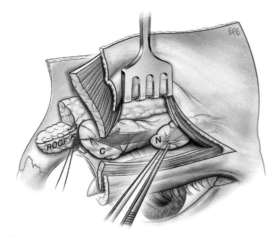

Fig. 5. Illustration showing the fat shifting technique. C, central fat pad; N, nasal fat pad. (*Courtesy of* Levent Efe, Brunswick, AU.)

compartment should not be surgically entered to keep the tissue planes intact for grafting. Fat grafting the ROOF is one component of enhancing the C-angle along with the suborbicularis oculi fat compartment. The central and medial upper lid fold are another target area for fat grafting particularly in secondary cases and in the presence of an A-frame deformity. The fat aliquots are placed using a 19F or 20F gauge cannula under the orbicularis oculi muscle. Fat grafting volume ranges from 1.5 to 3 mL per side depending on the area treated. Similarly, if fat grafting is planned to the upper lid fold, the tissue planes should be left undisrupted. This is more suited in cases where

the nasal fat pad is targeted through a small orbicularis window for excision while the remaining upper lid fold is volumize through fat grafting rather than orbital fat manipulation.

SUMMARY

The brow forms the aesthetic frame of the upper eyelid and brow lifting is a powerful maneuver to aesthetically shape and lateralize the curvature of the brow arc. Furthermore, brow lifting directly influences the upper eyelid fold height and the curvature of the upper eyelid crease. Careful aesthetic analysis, keeping in mind the aesthetic harmony of the upper periorbital arcs, is critical to optimize results given the varied presenting aging patterns of prospective patients. The surgeon must maintain a high index of suspicion of blepharoptosis and understand that combining complimentary procedures including ptosis repair, brow lift, upper periorbital fat shifting/contouring and fat grafting, as indicated, can help optimize outcomes by attaining a balanced result.

CLINICS CARE POINTS

- When evaluating a brow shape one should pay attention to the presence of blepharoptosis, which results in medial frontalis muscle strain and elevation of the medial brow resulting in medialization of the brow peak.

- When shaping the brow, one should distribute the fat volume and contour the muscle to achieve the ideal surface topography.

DISCLOSURE STATEMENT

The authors have nothing to disclose.

REFERENCES

1. Alghoul MS, Bricker JT, Venkatesh V, et al. Rethinking upper blepharoplasty: the impact of pretarsal show. Plast Reconstr Surg 2020;146(6): 1239–47.
2. Alghoul MS, Vaca EE, Mioton LM. Getting good results in cosmetic blepharoplasty. Plast Reconstr Surg 2020;146(1):71e–82e.
3. Vaca EE, Alghoul MS. Upper blepharoplasty with endoscopically assisted brow lift to restore

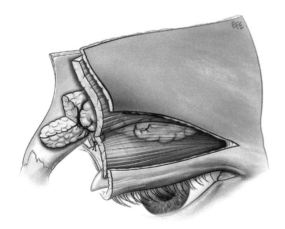

Fig. 6. Illustration showing the orbicularis oculi muscle to arcus marginalis suture for muscle and upper lid fold contouring. (*Courtesy of* Levent Efe, Brunswick, AU.)

harmonious upper lid arc curvatures. Plast Reconstr Surg 2020;146(5):565e–8e.

4. Turin SY, Vaca EE, Cheesborough JE, et al. Simplified lateral brow lift under local anesthesia for correction of lateral hooding. Plast Reconstr Surg Glob Open 2019;7(6):e2098.

5. Fagien S. Eyebrow analysis after blepharoplasty in patients with brow ptosis. Ophthalmic Plast Reconstr Surg 1992;8(3):210–4.

6. Fagien S. Advanced rejuvenative upper blepharoplasty: enhancing aesthetics of the upper periorbita. Plast Reconstr Surg 2002;110(1):278–91 [discussion: 292].

7. Siegel RJ, Fagien S. Seeking simplicity: golf tips and blepharoplasty. Plast Reconstr Surg 2003;112(1):343.

8. Rohrich RJ, Coberly DM, Fagien S, et al. Current concepts in aesthetic upper blepharoplasty. Plast Reconstr Surg 2004;113(3):32e–42e.

9. Fagien S. The role of the orbicularis oculi muscle and the eyelid crease in optimizing results in aesthetic upper blepharoplasty: a new look at the surgical treatment of mild upper eyelid fissure and fold asymmetries. Plast Reconstr Surg 2010;125(2):653–66.

10. Flowers RS, Flowers SS. Precision planning in blepharoplasty. The importance of preoperative mapping. Clin Plast Surg 1993;20(2):303–10.

11. Flowers RS. Upper blepharoplasty by eyelid invagination. Anchor blepharoplasty. Clin Plast Surg 1993;20(2):193–207.

12. Knize DM. Limited-incision forehead lift for eyebrow elevation to enhance upper blepharoplasty. Plast Reconstr Surg 1996;97(7):1334–42.

13. Knize DM. Limited incision forehead lift for eyebrow elevation to enhance upper blepharoplasty. Plast Reconstr Surg 2001;108(2):564–7.

14. Guyuron B, Knize DM. Corrugator supercilii resection through blepharoplasty incision. Plast Reconstr Surg 2001;107(2):606–7.

15. Guyuron B, Michelow BJ, Thomas T. Corrugator supercilii muscle resection through blepharoplasty incision. Plast Reconstr Surg 1995;95(4):691–6.

16. Guyuron B, Michelow BJ. Refinements in endoscopic forehead rejuvenation. Plast Reconstr Surg 1997;100(1):154–60.

17. Behmand RA, Guyuron B. Endoscopic forehead rejuvenation: II. Long-term results. Plast Reconstr Surg 2006;117(4):1137–43 [discussion: 1144].

18. Rowe DJ, Guyuron B. Optimizing results in endoscopic forehead rejuvenation. Clin Plast Surg 2008;35(3):355–60 [discussion: 353].

19. McCord CD Jr. Techniques in blepharoplasty. Ophthalmic Surg 1979;10(3):40–55.

20. McCord CD, Doxanas MT. Browplasty and browpexy: an adjunct to blepharoplasty. Plast Reconstr Surg 1990;86(2):248–54.

21. DiFrancesco LM, Anjema CM, Codner MA, et al. Evaluation of conventional subciliary incision used in blepharoplasty: preoperative and postoperative videography and electromyography findings. Plast Reconstr Surg 2005;116(2):632–9.

22. Vaca EE, Bricker JT, Helenowski I, et al. Identifying aesthetically appealing upper eyelid topographic proportions. Aesthet Surg J 2019;39(8):824–34.

23. Vaca EE, Purnell CA, Gosain AK, et al. Postoperative temporal hollowing: is there a surgical approach that prevents this complication? A systematic review and anatomic illustration. J Plast Reconstr Aesthet Surg 2017;70(3):401–15.

24. Agarwal CA, Mendenhall SD 3rd, Foreman KB, et al. The course of the frontal branch of the facial nerve in relation to fascial planes: an anatomic study. Plast Reconstr Surg 2010;125(2):532–7.

25. Alghoul M, Codner MA. Retaining ligaments of the face: review of anatomy and clinical applications. Aesthet Surg J 2013;33(6):769–82.

26. Moss CJ, Mendelson BC, Taylor GI. Surgical anatomy of the ligamentous attachments in the temple and periorbital regions. Plast Reconstr Surg 2000;105(4):1475–90 [discussion: 1491-1478].

27. Hargiss JL. Surgical anatomy of the eyelids. Trans Pac Coast Otoophthalmol Soc Annu Meet 1963;44:193–202.

28. Muzaffar AR, Mendelson BC, Adams WP Jr. Surgical anatomy of the ligamentous attachments of the lower lid and lateral canthus. Plast Reconstr Surg 2002;110(3):873–84 [discussion: 897-911].

29. Kikkawa DO, Lemke BN, Dortzbach RK. Relations of the superficial musculoaponeurotic system to the orbit and characterization of the orbitomalar ligament. Ophthalmic Plast Reconstr Surg 1996;12(2):77–88.

30. Wong CH, Hsieh MKH, Mendelson B. The tear trough ligament: anatomical basis for the tear trough deformity. Plast Reconstr Surg 2012;129(6):1392–402.

31. Hwang K, Nam YS, Kim DJ, et al. Surgical anatomy of retaining ligaments in the periorbital area. J Craniofac Surg 2008;19(3):800–4.

32. Ghavami A, Pessa JE, Janis J, et al. The orbicularis retaining ligament of the medial orbit: closing the circle. Plast Reconstr Surg 2008;121(3):994–1001.

33. Knize DM. The superficial lateral canthal tendon: anatomic study and clinical application to lateral canthopexy. Plast Reconstr Surg 2002;109(3):1149–57 [discussion: 1158-1163].

34. Christensen KN, Lachman N, Pawlina W, et al. Cutaneous depth of the supraorbital nerve: a cadaveric anatomic study with clinical applications to dermatology. Dermatol Surg 2014;40(12):1342–8.

35. Janis JE, Ghavami A, Lemmon JA, et al. The anatomy of the corrugator supercilii muscle: part II.

Supraorbital nerve branching patterns. Plast Reconstr Surg 2008;121(1):233–40.

36. Trussler AP, Stephan P, Hatef D, et al. The frontal branch of the facial nerve across the zygomatic arch: anatomical relevance of the high-SMAS technique. Plast Reconstr Surg 2010;125(4):1221–9.

37. Trinei FA, Januszkiewicz J, Nahai F. The sentinel vein: an important reference point for surgery in the temporal region. Plast Reconstr Surg 1998; 101(1):27–32.

38. Alghoul MS, Vaca EE, Bricker JT, et al. Enhancing the lateral orbital "C-angle" with calcium hydroxylapatite: an anatomic and clinical study. Aesthet Surg J 2021;41(8):952–66.

39. Massry GG. Nasal fat preservation in upper eyelid blepharoplasty. Ophthalmic Plast Reconstr Surg 2011;27(5):352–5.

40. Zarem HA, Resnick JI, Carr RM, et al. Browpexy: lateral orbicularis muscle fixation as an adjunct to upper blepharoplasty. Plast Reconstr Surg 1997; 100(5):1258–61.

41. Ramil ME. Fat grafting in hollow upper eyelids and volumetric upper blepharoplasty. Plast Reconstr Surg 2017;140(5):889–97.

Noninvasive Correction of the Aging Forehead

Malcolm P. Chelliah, MD, MBA*, Shilpi Khetarpal, MD

KEYWORDS

• Upper face • Rejuvenation • Noninvasive • Forehead • Brows

KEY POINTS

- Aging of the upper face occurs in many ways including loss of bone, fat, and skin laxity.
- Combination therapy is ideal to achieve the best results.
- Good patient selection is critical when offering nonsurgical interventions, as some patients may be expecting surgical results with noninvasive procedures.
- A thorough understanding of facial anatomy is crucial for safety.

INTRODUCTION

As has previously been discussed, aging of the face is a continuous and dynamic process that occurs due to changes in layers including skin, muscle, fat, and bone. There is an increasing patient preference toward nonsurgical techniques and procedures that require minimal downtime in all aspects of cosmetic surgery. The periorbital region is no exception.

The mainstay of treatment involves the administration of injectable fillers for temple volumization, eyebrow reshaping and forehead contouring, and neuromodulation to reduce the appearance of dynamic rhytids. In addition, judicious weakening of the brow depressor muscles using botulinum toxin can result in lateral brow elevation and widening the eye. These 2 approaches can be combined for an optimal cosmetic appearance. During the same visit it is recommended to inject filler first followed by injection of neuromodulator. However, if the visits are spaced apart, neuromodulator injection should be first used to address any dynamic rhytids and filler to address any static concerns at subsequent visits.

Surgical and nonsurgical procedures can be used in combination in order to maximize periorbital rejuvenation. This article focuses on nonsurgical rejuvenation of the brow and periorbital complex. Surgical correction is addressed in ensuing articles.

EVALUATION

Although the focus of this article is the upper third of the face, a full assessment of the face and complete understanding of the relationships between muscles is paramount for optimal success. In addition, it is vital to assess the patient's appearance in both its natural resting state and with maximum facial motion. Take note whether there be any existing facial asymmetries that will require refinement of the treatment technique; this is important because once movement has been blocked, one must anticipate extra movement elsewhere, which may require treatment. Equally as important is noting whether the patient persistently uses the frontalis muscle to lift the brow, as relaxation of the frontalis with toxin will inadvertently lead to unwanted brow ptosis. Modulation of the frontalis muscle will then need to be tempered in order to avoid this outcome.

Dermatochalasis may also result from relaxation of the frontalis muscle and give the appearance of a swollen or heavy upper eyelid. Often this is only discovered after treatment in which case upper eyelid surgery is needed for best correction.

An understanding of the patient's prior cosmetic treatments is beneficial as well. For example, previous browlift or blepharoplasty should be noted as should previous neuromodulator or filler treatment. Patient satisfaction with previous treatment, dosage, and treatment

Department of Dermatology, Cleveland Clinic Foundation, 2049 East 100th Street, Cleveland, OH 44195, USA
* Corresponding author.
E-mail address: chellim@ccf.org

Clin Plastic Surg 49 (2022) 399–407
https://doi.org/10.1016/j.cps.2022.03.004
0094-1298/22/© 2022 Elsevier Inc. All rights reserved.

location should be noted. The timing of any of these treatments can affect the patient's expectations. A thorough understanding of the patient's goal is required so that overtreatment does not yield an undesirable outcome and maintains a natural, refreshed look. It is always possible to add more at a later visit. However, with overadministration patient dissatisfaction is prolonged for the duration of the neuromodulator effect. Of course all botulinum effect, good or bad, is temporary. In general, men have stronger muscles and may require more neurotoxin. Men are more likely to desire some movement after injection. Patients with regular maintenance schedules will require fewer units with time, as their muscles weaken from repeated administration. With discontinuation of treatment, previous muscle mass and tone is restored.

Although a detailed anatomy review is beyond the scope of this article, a basic understanding is crucial while performing facial rejuvenation. The glabellar subunit is composed of 2 corrugator supercilii muscles and the procerus muscle that contracts to pull the brow both medially and downward. The corrugator supercilii are typically medial to the midpupillary line; however, in some patients it may extend beyond this and can be assessed during maximal frowning. Contraction of these glabellar muscles produce the vertically oriented rhytides between the brows. The medial aspect of the frontalis muscle coalesces with the glabellar subunit and the lateral portion with the lateral aspect of orbicularis oculi. The main function of the vertically oriented frontalis is to elevate the brow and upper eyelids. Its contraction causes linearly oriented rhytids across the forehead. The frontalis muscle terminates laterally at the superior temporal line. Therefore, lateral to this landmark there is no elevator muscle present; this is important because the lateral orbicularis therefore acts unopposed, and this is the primary reason that the lateral brow descends with age. The levator palpebrae muscle lies just beneath the orbicularis oculi and serves to elevate the upper eyelid.

Photography is beneficial and demonstrating progress the patient has made through their aesthetic journey. There is only one opportunity to take a proper "before" photo, and this will be used as the baseline with which "after" photos are compared. It is wise to have all photos standardized and taken with the same camera and lighting conditions to reduce variables as much as possible. It is also advisable to take photos at rest and with muscle contraction before performing neurotoxin injections.

NEUROTOXIN

Neurotoxins produced by the bacteria *Clostridium botulinum* inhibit the release of acetylcholine at the presynaptic neuromuscular junction, resulting in a localized reduction of the function of the muscle. The effect usually begins over the first 7 days and generally from 3 to 4 months. For clinical purposes, the main serotypes are A and B, with serotype A (BTA) most frequently used for cosmetic indications such as onabotulinumtoxinA (Botox Cosmetic; Allergan, Irvine, CA, USA), incobotulinumtoxinA (Dysport; Medicis, Scottsdale, AZ, USA), and abobotulinumtoxinA (Xeomin; Merz Aesthetics, San Mateo, CA, USA), which are all Food and Drug Administration (FDA) approved to treat rhytides. Botox, Dysport, and Xeomin each differ slightly based on accessory proteins or lack thereof as is the case of Xeomin. In general, it is provider preference which version is used for patients. Rimabotulinum-toxin B (Myobloc; Soltice Neurosciences Inc, San Francisco, CA, USA) is FDA approved for the treatment of cervical dystonia. This product is also used off-label in nonresponders to serotype A of the toxin.

Botulinum toxins are consistently effective in the treatment of dynamic lines such as those caused by corrugator hyperactivity (**Fig. 1**). Patients should be made aware that the administration of neurotoxin will not improve the appearance of static lines that are unrelated to facial muscle contraction. In addition, it will not improve excess or sagging skin, and patients expecting such dramatic outcomes are likely best served with a surgical options.

The glabella is the primary FDA-approved indication for treatment of rhytids with BTA. Treatment typically involves injection of the procerus, 2 injections to the depressor supercilii bilaterally and 2 into the corrugators bilaterally with a total range of 10 to 30 units for the entire aesthetic unit.

The orbital portion of the orbicularis oculi also depresses the brow, and consequently, the presence of crow's feet leads to lowering of the lateral aspect of the brow as well. Eyebrow lifting can be achieved through a series of neurotoxin administrations of 2.5 to 5 units of OnaBoNT-A to the lateral aspects of the orbicularis oculi muscle with the superior of these at approximately 0.5 cm inferior and lateral to the tail of the brow.

SOFT TISSUE AUGMENTATION

Age-related volume loss and atrophy can be counteracted through the administration of temporary injectable fillers. In addition to restoring lost volume, fillers can reduce rhytides, restore skin laxity, and achieve facial contouring.

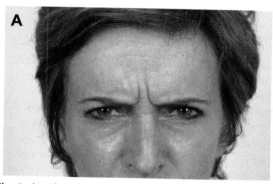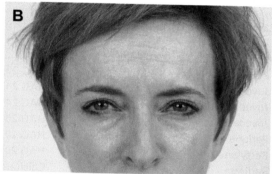

Fig. 1. (*A, B*) A 53-year-old woman activating corrugator muscle. (*A*) Before injection of 10 units of botulinum A into each corrugator muscle and 5 units in the procerus for a total of 25 units. (*Courtesy of* James Zins, MD, Cleveland, OH.)

As with neurotoxin administration, patient selection is critical in obtaining a successful cosmetic outcome. Patients with volume loss–related bone resorption and fat redistribution are better candidates for fillers than those with significant skin laxity or skin that has been weathered with extreme sun exposure. Contraindication to filler placement includes pregnancy, active infection at the potential site of injection, allergy to products, and recent or upcoming dental work or any procedure that might shed bacteria into the bloodstream.[1] During the consultation, a thorough review of medical history is recommended. In particular, the use of prescription and/or over-the-counter vitamins and supplements that are known blood thinners such as aspirin or garlic, ginseng, and vitamin E should be ascertained.[2] To minimize postprocedure bruising, these should all be discontinued 1 week before injection. However, this is not always practical, and injection with patients on antiplatelet drugs offer minimal risk. Moderate amount of alcohol consumption has also been reported to inhibit platelet activation, leading to bruising, and patients should be counseled to avoid drinking both before (approximately 48 hours prior) and after the procedure. Certain medical disorders such as those involving collagen, scarring or connective tissue, lupus, and recent treatment with isotretinoin may have a contraindication as well.[3,4]

There are a wide variety of filler options, and most of them are temporary. Of these, most are reversible owing to composition of hyaluronic acid gel (HAG), which can be reversed with hyaluronidase. In addition, HA is the most abundant glycosaminoglycan in the skin and consequently has a minimal allergic reaction potential. Hyaluronic acid (HA) gel products differ based on various properties such as cross-linking and HA concentration, which affects their rheologic characteristics. Other filler options include calcium hydroxyapatite, fat grafting, permanent soft tissue filler, and poly-L-lactic acid. In the injectable naïve patient, options for filler that are reversible and temporary are generally preferred.

The location of filler injection offers some influence in the option chosen due to the difference in rheologic characteristics, which determines the flow of the gel.[5] G prime (G′) is a measurement of the stiffness of the HAG and determines how well the gel opposes distortion. Higher levels of G′ correspond to greater resistance to distortion, which is useful in scenarios where lift is required. Viscosity defines the ability to either remain localized at the site of injection or to diffuse out into the surrounding tissues. A lower viscosity filler also takes less force to inject and flows easily into the skin, allowing for more molding afterward. Cohesivity is a measure of the gel's cross-linking and determines how well the gel sticks together without spreading apart. Lower cohesive fillers will conform more easily to bone, whereas fillers with higher cohesivity will maintain its shape better. Monophasic fillers are homogenous and have a higher cohesivity, whereas biphasic fillers contain microspheres of various sizes and have a lower cohesivity. A summary of the characteristics of fillers is provided in **Table 1**.

Exact injection techniques will differ based on the type of filler used, area of filler, and the experience of the injector. In general, underfilling is better than overfilling. The primary techniques for injecting filler are vertical surpraperiosteal depot, tower technique, serial puncture, linear threading, fanning, and cross-hatching. Serial puncture or linear threading is ideal for filling the glabella and/or fine lines in the forehead. A combination of both techniques, serially puncturing the skin with short anterograde or retrograde injections tends toward optimal results. For larger areas such as

Table 1
A summary of the characteristics of fillers

Product	Manufacturer	Type	G′	Reversible	Duration
Belotero Balance	Merz	HAG 22.5 mg/mL	39	Yes	12 mo
Juvéderm Ultra	Allergan	HAG 24 mg/mL	94	Yes	12 mo
Juvéderm Ultra Plus	Allergan	HAG 24 mg/mL	135	Yes	18 mo
Juvéderm Voluma	Allergan	HAG 20 mg/mL	270	Yes	6–9 mo
Perlane	Galderma	HAG 20 mg/mL	541	Yes	6–9 mo
Restylane	Galderma	HAG 20 mg/mL	864	Yes	6–9 mo
Radiesse	Merz	Calcium hydroxyapatite	1407	No	12–15 mo
Sculptra	Aventis	Poly-L-lactic acid	NA	No	1–2 y
Bellafill	Suneva Medical	Polymethylmethacrylate	NA	No	5–10 y

Abbreviations: G′, viscous modulus; HAG, hyaluronic acid gel; NA, not applicable.

inflating the concavity of the forehead, cross-hatching or fanning is effective. For cross-hatching, a series of linear threads are injected in parallel followed by another series of injection in parallel but together are perpendicular to the first series, thereby forming a progressive grid. Fanning is performed by inserting the needle in a single insertion point and radially injecting filler in a clockwise or counterclockwise fashion.

Before injecting, palpate the area to ensure it is not overlying an arterial pulse. Although it has been previously thought that aspiration before injection can alert the injector to danger, additional studies have shown that this should not be relied on as a safety maneuver due to the possibility of a false negative.[6] Instead, it is best to minimize injections of large boluses into a localized area in favor of smaller, microboluses with constant needle movement and low extrusion pressure. The amount of filler placed will depend on the amount of volume lost. Large-diameter blunt cannulas (22 or 25 gauge) may reduce the risk of intravascular injection and may also reduce the risk of bleeding. However, this comment is controversial, and their use is not failsafe.

Volume loss in the glabella, forehead, and brow contributes to an aged appearance in the upper face. The ideal female brow aesthetics has trended toward a lower and flatter brow, with the peak lying at the lateral third of the brow or at the lateral canthus.[7] A youthful female forehead is slightly convex, 12° off vertical.[8] To expand any supra brow concavity, the authors recommend a highly cohesive, low G′ filler that spreads in the subgaleal plane along the periosteum below the level of the frontalis at the midprocerus level between the supratrochlear vascular arteries. A slow and gentle anterograde injection technique with radial fanning followed by gently massaging

the area will ensure an even dispersion minimizing lumps.[9] This additional support along the periosteum allows the frontalis to relax, leading to softening of the horizontal forehead lines. Avoid the supratrochlear and supraorbital arteries that lie in this area. The supraorbital vessels exit the supraorbital notch, which is readily palpable and is approximately 25 mm from the midline. The supratrochlear vessel is 8 to 12 mm medial to the supraorbital vessel and is easily identified by asking the patient to frown, as it is found directly under the glabellar creases.

In contrast to the forehead, if filler is needed to fill any defects in the glabellar subunit, it is important to inject in the dermis and not subdermally to avoid intravascular injection. The injection "danger zones" are located in the central face, as this is where the large vessels lie.

When administering filler to enhance brow contour, injections should be placed conservatively so as to prevent the development of a heavy brow. Care should also be taken to avoid the orbital branch of the superficial temporal artery that anastomoses with the supraorbital artery just above the brow. Inject 0.25 to 0.5 mL of filler along the supraorbital ridge, entering approximately 1 cm lateral to and 0.5 cm inferior to the point at which the parietal suture crosses the orbital ridge. The filler injection should be tapered to minimize the transition between the treated and the untreated areas, with the maximum volume of filler placed deep to the lateral third of the brow.

Injection of filler into the temples can help reduce skeletonized shadowing, resulting in a more youthful facial appearance. Reinflating the temple can also help achieve lateral brow elevation. Injection deep to the temporalis muscle just above periosteum is the safe depth for injection in this area and minimizes the risk of contact with

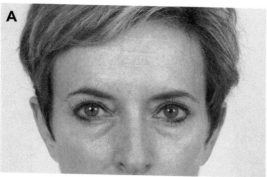
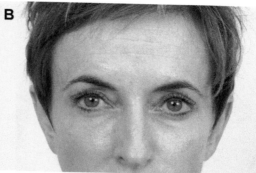

Fig. 2. (*A, B*) A 53-year-old woman with lower lid bags. (*A*) Before soft tissue augmentation with 0.5 cc of Restylane per lid. (*B*) One month following injection of 0. 5 cc of Restylane per lid. (*Courtesy of* James Zins, MD, Cleveland, OH.)

the anterior branch of the superficial temporal artery that anastomoses with the supraorbital artery in the subdermal plane. Filler should be placed 1 cm above the zygomatic arch, which minimizes the risk of injecting into the middle temporal vein located superficially in the subcutaneous space; intravascular injection into this area could result in blindness.[10,11]

The superior medial quadrant of the orbit resorbs with age and loss of this support contributes to eyelid ptosis. In these patients, assess whether the frontalis muscle is being used to compensate for eyelid ptosis; this will lead to deep horizontal rhytids in the forehead, and filling the superior medial quadrant of the orbit to minimize ptosis can allow for relaxation of the frontalis muscle via neurotoxin to improve the appearance in both areas. To fill the orbit, inject midline of the forehead approximately 1 cm superior to the nasal root with a maximum of 0.5 mL per side. The depth of injection should be around the level of the orbicularis muscle but superficial to the bone, as there are large arteries at the periosteal level that should be avoided. The needle should be kept away from the globe of the eye. In the periorbital area, temporary and reversible HAG fillers are preferred (**Fig. 2**).

Other investigators such as Pavicic and colleagues[12] have described a multistep process to facial rejuvenation by first relaxing muscles with BTA followed by injection of calcium hydroxyapatite 4 weeks later and then finally hyaluronic acid 2 to 4 weeks after hydroxyapatite injection. The overall goal was to restore youth and reinflate defects and lines without overcorrection. In the eyebrow area typically Restylane or Juvéderm Ultra are used: in the upper eyelid sulcus area dilute Restylane or Juvéderm Ultra and in the lower eyelid area typically Restylane or Belotero (**Fig. 3**). The choice of HA filler used in each area

depends on the concentration of the HAG, which affects how hydrophilic the gel is. Higher concentrations correspond to a more hydrophilic gel, which draws more fluid into the area. This property can be used to augment the upper eyelid superior sulcus deformity but can cause excess fluid retention such as in the lower eyelid hollows. The authors prefer Restylane rather than Juvéderm in the tear trough/lower lid area because the hydrophilic nature of Juvéderm can lead to overcorrection in this area.

DEVICES
Lasers and Light Emitting Devices

There are several laser and light emitting devices that can be used to tighten the skin of the brow and the upper eyelid.[13] Nonablative options include erbium midinfrared, infrared, and near-infrared lasers. Ablative options include fractionated carbon dioxide and fractionated erbium:YAG lasers. These options can stimulate collagenesis and/or elastogenesis, creating true structural changes in the treated area. Devices that touch the mid to deep dermis and the hypodermis are more likely to create longer lasting changes with the general consensus being that CO_2 laser ablation is superior to Er:YAG ablation with regard to creating tissue contraction and improvement in rhytides[14] (**Fig. 4**).

Radiofrequency and Ultrasound

Owing to the long wavelength of radiofrequency (RF), these devices are able to heat the dermis and the hypodermis between 45 and 65° C to stimulate existing dermal collagen fibers and neocollagenesis. Fractional bipolar RF heats the dermis volumetrically independent of a targeted chromophore. Positively and negatively charged electrodes deliver the RF energy through the

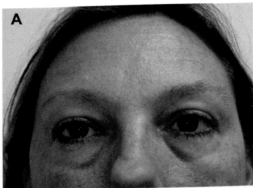
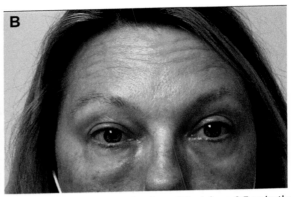

Fig. 3. (*A*, *B*) A 46-year-old Caucasian woman with lower lid bags. (*A*) Before injection of Restylane 0.5 cc in the right and 0.5 cc in the left lower lid tear trough region. (*B*) Two months following injection.

epidermis and dermis and form a closed circuit loop of RF current. Most of the energy delivered passes through the epidermis and targets the dermis directly due to the higher concentration of water and electrolytes compared with the epidermis, resulting in limited epidermal ablation but allowing for ablative resurfacing.[15] In addition, the energy is delivered in an inverted conical shape focusing on the effect on the dermis. Because of this, these devices can safely be used on all Fitzpatrick skin types including type VI. Multiple single passes can be performed to provide upward and outward vectoring effect at the temples and superolateral mid-face before treatment of the full face, including the forehead, with sublative resurfacing.

Device settings vary depending on the depth of ablative zones; the extent of surrounding coagulated tissue; and the proportions of coagulation, necrosis, and ablation. RF energy of up to 62 mJ per electrode pin can be delivered, with coagulation and necrosis up to a maximum depth of approximately 450 μm and epidermal ablation of 5% to 7%.[16] The number of electrode pins on the tip can also be varied. For a given RF fluence, the smaller the number of pins, the greater the depth of penetration of the closed loops of RF current.

In addition to bipolar devices, there are also multisource phase-controlled RF devices that use multiple electrodes and RF generators, continuous monopolar RF that is useful for subdermal heating, combined monopolar and bipolar RF that can simultaneously deliver deep and superficial volumetric heating, and fractional bipolar RF that delivers energy via an array of microneedles.

Microfocused Ultrasound

Microfocused ultrasound (MFU) can help to improve thinner rhytids through delivering discreet foci of microthermal coagulation deeper into tissues. Ulthera is currently the only device cleared for nonsurgical brow lifting. Ultrasound energy at

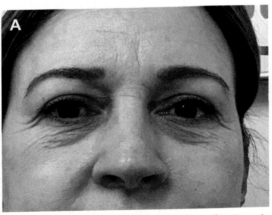
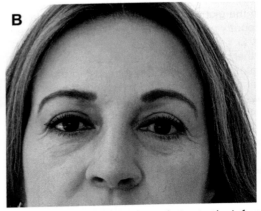

Fig. 4. (*A*, *B*) A 56-year-old Hispanic woman after 2 sessions of fractional ablative CO2 resurfacing to the infraorbital region. (*A*) Pretreatment. (*B*) Eight months posttreatment.

a frequency of 4 to 7 MHz is delivered to focused discreet zones inducing microcoagulation within the dermis and hypodermis. The depth can be adjusted to reach the subcutaneous muscular aponeurotic system while sparing the epidermis.[17] While using the device, there is simultaneous imaging of the tissue planes being targeted; this is similar to the RF devices. The resulting thermal energy causes collagen contracture, creating a lifting effect and stimulates neocollagenesis while sparing the epidermis.[18] Because of this sparing, MFU devices can be safely used in all skin types with minimal risk of postinflammatory hyperpigmentation. For lifting of the eyebrows, the device is applied to the lateral part of the forehead, including the region just above the lateral two-thirds of the eyebrows, and MFU energy is delivered at a depth of 3 mm.

COMPLICATIONS/CONCERNS

Acute or subacute infection may present with erythema, edema, and tenderness. While infections are uncommon, there is a rare risk of biofilm formation, and as such, systemic antibiotics are first-line treatment. Other measures such as incision and drainage or removal of the filler via hyaluronidase may be required. The best measure to prevent infection is to cleanse the face thoroughly before injection, avoid filling through the oral or nasal mucosa, and not injecting into traumatized skin.

Ecchymosis and temporary tenderness or swelling may occur after filler or neurotoxin administration. Cool compresses or ice packs used before and after injections can be used to minimize any discomfort. Mild ecchymosis can respond to topical vitamin K cream.[19] Significant ecchymoses can be treated with pulse dye laser to accelerate recovery. Observe for tenderness and fluctuance, which may be a sign of an underlying hematoma.

Contour irregularities can result when filling convexities. These are best minimized through avoiding overfilling. Remember, additional amounts of filler can always be added later. Minor irregularities can be improved by tissue molding after injection. Any unwanted HAG can be dissolved with hyaluronidase diluted with lidocaine.

Nodules may occur after filler administration and may be either inflammatory of noninflammatory in nature. Most cases of noninflammatory nodules are the result of poor filler injection technique, that is, from overfilling or too superficial placement.[20] The use of particulate fillers in highly dynamic areas such as the lips can lead to a delayed onset nodule formation. Early appearing nodules may respond to firm massage with or without preceding lidocaine or saline administration.[21] Nodules with HA filler will resolve with hyaluronidase; however, non-HA filler may require small amounts of intralesional steroids. Patients should also continue massage at home to disrupt any nodules. Nodules that fail to resolve may require excision as a last resort.

Although most long-standing inflammatory nodules are foreign body granulomas, any time there is a persistent red, indurated nodule, biofilm formation should be suspected. As such, antibiotic treatment should be the first step. It is important to be aware that biofilm formation is usually culture negative, and confirmation may require either fluorescence in situ hybridization[22] or the use of scintigraphy with radiolabeled autologous white blood cells.[23] The exact incidence of biofilm formation following filler administration is unknown and diagnosis is difficult; however, fortunately this remains a rare complication. Foreign body granulomas are also rare with an estimated incidence between 0.01% and 1%.[4] There is usually a latency period anywhere from several months to years following injection. Over time, these lesions become firmer due to the development of fibrosis. The shape of microspheres seems to influence the development of granulomas with reactions occurring less frequently with smaller, smoother microspheres.

Pigmentary alteration can be a concern in all skin types but in particular in Fitzpatrick skin types IV to VI. The most common occurrence is at the site of injection. Mild hyperpigmentation should fade with time and ample use of sunscreen. Additions of topical hydroquinone and/or Retin-A can speed the process or be used in more moderate to severe cases. Resistant postinflammatory hyperpigmentation can be treated with chemical or low-fluence ND:YAG 1064 nm laser.

In lighter skin types, injection of filler into the superficial dermis or epidermis can inadvertently leave a bluish hue as a result of the Tyndall effect. This effect is worsened with more superficial injections of filler. Dissolution with hyaluronidase should be the first step; if there is any remainder due to a high degree of cross-linking or large particle size, then expression of the unwanted filler may be achieved by a small incision.

Major Complications

The danger of intravascular filler injection can be headed off with a thorough understanding of facial anatomy and through injecting the correct filler at the appropriate tissue level to avoid major neurovascular bundles. As previously discussed, drawing back on the syringe is not an efficient method of determining an entry into a vessel. Injecting small boluses slowly can help to minimize the risk of intravascular injection. It is better to select a higher G' filler to create a lifting affect than to inject large boluses. Large boluses of filler also increase the risk of filler migration. Vascular complications are at highest risk when injecting filler in the midline, the so called "danger zone." Inadvertent intravascular injection can result in a filler embolus and vascular occlusion of end vessels. The first signs of this include pain out of proportion to the injection area as well as blanching. Five hundred units Hyaluronidase per aesthetic unit should be administered immediately and continued every hour until complete resolution has occurred serially until blood flow is restored. Although this is an emergency, the physician has hours or even days to reverse the threatened tissue loss; this is in contradistinction to visual loss due to filler injection when minutes now become critical. Visual loss occurs when the internal carotid system (supraorbital or supratrochlear artery) is inadvertently entered and filler is injected under pressure. Retrograde bolus of filler enters the ophthalmic or retinal artery. When syringe pressure is released filler enters the ophthalmic or retinal artery and an antegrade filler embolus results.

Laser Complications

Patients treated with fractionated ablative lasers are also at risk of developing secondary infections from either bacteria or viral outbreaks from herpes. Signs of secondary infection include erythema, tenderness, and purulence as well as vesicles in the case of herpes. If there is any suspicion, obtain cultures and start empirical systemic antibiotics or antivirals. Rarely, Candida can colonize the skin after treatment, leading to persistent facial erythema and pustules that are refractory to typical antibiotic treatment.

CLINICS CARE POINTS

- It is essential when evaluating a patient to find out their primary concerns and goals. Noninvasive and minimally invasive techniques can be effective for subtle improvement, but patients looking for near full correction would be best suited with surgery followed by injectables to maintain improvement.
- Photography is also an essential part of the consultation, ensuring standardized lighting,

positioning, and making sure the patient does not have makeup on. The duration of each product being used and the expectation for future treatments should also be stressed.

- Given the fat, skin, and bones change in many ways, combination therapy is ideal when deciding on a treatment plan for not just the upper face, but when treating any portion of the face and neck.

DISCLOSURE

The authors have no direct financial interest in subject matter or materials discussed in this article or with a company making a competing product.

REFERENCES

1. De Boulle K, Heydenrych I. Patient factors influencing dermal filler complications: prevention, assessment, and treatment. Clin Cosmet Investig Dermatol 2015;8:205–14.
2. Dinehart SM, Henry L. Dietary supplements: altered coagulation and effects on bruising. Dermatol Surg 2005;31(7 Pt 2):819–26 [discussion: 826].
3. Creadore A, Watchmaker J, Maymone MBC, et al. Cosmetic treatment in patients with autoimmune connective tissue diseases: best practices for patients with lupus erythematosus. J Am Acad Dermatol 2020;83(2):343–63.
4. Funt D, Pavicic T. Dermal fillers in aesthetics: an overview of adverse events and treatment approaches. Clin Cosmet Investig Dermatol 2013;6: 295–316.
5. Sundaram H, Cassuto D. Biophysical characteristics of hyaluronic acid soft-tissue fillers and their relevance to aesthetic applications. Plast Reconstr Surg 2013;132(4 Suppl 2):5S–21S.
6. Moon HJ, Lee W, Kim JS, et al. Aspiration revisited: prospective evaluation of a physiologically pressurized model with animal correlation and broader applicability to filler complications. Aesthetic Surg J 2021;41(8):NP1073–83.
7. Griffin GR, Kim JC. Ideal female brow aesthetics. Clin Plast Surg 2013;40(1):147–55.
8. Goodman GJ. The oval female facial shape–a study in beauty. Dermatol Surg 2015;41(12):1375–83.
9. Narins RS, Donofrio LM. Unique injection techniques, including volumizing the forehead, advance the ways we rejuvenate the face. Dermatol Surg 2010;36(Suppl 3):1799.
10. Kapoor KM, Bertossi D, Li CQ, et al. A systematic literature review of the middle temporal vein anatomy: 'venous danger zone' in temporal fossa for filler injections. Aesthetic Plast Surg 2020;44(5):1803–10.

11. Jung W, Youn KH, Won SY, et al. Clinical implications of the middle temporal vein with regard to temporal fossa augmentation. Dermatol Surg 2014;40(6): 618–23.

12. Pavicic T, Few JW, Huber-Vorländer J. A novel, multi-step, combination facial rejuvenation procedure for treatment of the whole face with incobotulinumtox-inA, and two dermal fillers- calcium hydroxylapatite and a monophasic, polydensified hyaluronic acid filler. J Drugs Dermatol 2013;12(9):978–84.

13. Alexiades-Armenakas MR, Dover JS, Arndt KA. The spectrum of laser skin resurfacing: nonablative, frac-tional, and ablative laser resurfacing. J Am Acad Dermatol 2008;58(5):719–37. quiz 738-40.

14. Ross EV, Miller C, Meehan K, et al. One-pass CO2 versus multiple-pass Er:YAG laser resurfacing in the treatment of rhytides: a comparison side-by-side study of pulsed CO2 and Er:YAG lasers. Der-matol Surg 2001;27(8):709–15.

15. Friedman DJ, Gilead LT. The use of hybrid radiofre-quency device for the treatment of rhytides and lax skin. Dermatol Surg 2007;33(5):543–51.

16. Javate RM, Cruz RT, Khan J, et al. Nonablative 4-MHz dual radiofrequency wand rejuvenation treat-ment for periorbital rhytides and midface laxity. Ophthalmic Plast Reconstr Surg 2011;27(3):180–5.

17. White WM, Makin IR, Barthe PG, et al. Selective cre-ation of thermal injury zones in the superficial mus-culoaponeurotic system using intense ultrasound therapy: a new target for noninvasive facial rejuve-nation. Arch Facial Plast Surg 2007;9(1):22–9.

18. Alam M, White LE, Martin N, et al. Ultrasound tight-ening of facial and neck skin: a rater-blinded pro-spective cohort study. J Am Acad Dermatol 2010; 62(2):262–9.

19. Shah NS, Lazarus MC, Bugdodel R, et al. The ef-fects of topical vitamin K on bruising after laser treat-ment. J Am Acad Dermatol 2002;47(2):241–4.

20. Sclafani AP, Fagien S. Treatment of injectable soft tissue filler complications. Dermatol Surg 2009; 35(Suppl 2):1672–80.

21. Urdiales-Gálvez F, Delgado NE, Figueiredo V, et al. Treatment of soft tissue filler complications: expert consensus recommendations. Aesthet Plast Surg 2018;42(2):498–510.

22. Bjarnsholt T, Tolker-Nielsen T, Givskov M, et al. Detection of bacteria by fluorescence in situ hybrid-ization in culture-negative soft tissue filler lesions. Dermatol Surg 2009;35(Suppl 2):1620–4.

23. Grippaudo FR, Pacilio M, Di Girolamo M, et al. Ra-diolabelled white blood cell scintigraphy in the work-up of dermal filler complications. Eur J Nucl Med Mol Imaging 2013;40(3):418–25.

Direct Browlift

Julian D. Perry, MD*, Catherine J. Hwang, MD, FACS

KEYWORDS

- Brow ptosis • Browlift • Direct browlift • Frontalis muscle transposition browlift • Internal browlift

KEY POINTS

- Direct browlift represents a spectrum of surgeries to improve brow ptosis with incisions on or near the brow.
- These techniques can improve brow ptosis in a powerful and straightforward manner.
- Although direct browlift does leave visible scars, the scars can often be concealed in a cosmetically acceptable fashion and may represent the best option for selected patients depending on their anatomy, morphology, and commitment to surgery.

INTRODUCTION/HISTORY/DEFINITIONS/BACKGROUND

If incisions did not result in scars, then most surgical browlifts would directly lift the brows with incisions close to the target area for lifting. These techniques allow for rapid, predictable, and powerful elevation of the brows.

Unfortunately, despite our best efforts and technologies, incisions still do leave scars, especially in the multicontoured area of the brow, with its dense pilosebaceous units medially and thicker skin of approximately 1 to 1.3 mm. For this reason, efforts to conceal incisions in the hairline have been developed. Concealed incisions require more time, dissection, tissue disruption, risk of nerve and muscle damage, equipment, anesthesia, and cost.

The only reason to increase the amount of dissection is to attempt to conceal incisions. Thus, for patients in whom the incision cannot be concealed, it may not make sense to increase the surgical effort without significant benefit. Direct browlifting represents the most powerful way to lift an eyebrow, as it operates immediately on the area of regard. It is the most predictable option regarding the amount of lift, as it is directly proportional to the amount of tissue resected.

Direct browlifting is appropriate for individuals who desire an elevated brow and are not concerned about scarring, those who are not committed to the extra time, dissection, and/or cost of concealing the scar distant from the site of intended elevation, in some patients who do not have other areas to hide incisions, and in patients with severe asymmetry including paralytic brow ptosis.

EVALUATION

Normal brow position varies significantly, but the medial eyebrow is usually approximately 1 cm above the medial aspect of the superior orbital rim.[1] In women, a higher eyebrow arch is often present, with the apex of the arch located over the lateral limbus.[2] In men, the eyebrow often takes a flatter curve, is straighter, more diffuse, and located more inferiorly.[3,4] By manually raising the medial and lateral aspect of the eyebrow during an examination in a mirror, the normal anatomy as well as improvement of the tissue redundancies of the medial and lateral canthi can be demonstrated to the patient.

Patients with tattooed, microbladed, or painted brows require particular attention to determine and demonstrate to the patient the actual height of the brow rather than the brow cilia/pigment. Many patients have these tattoos placed higher than the actual eyebrow, and these patients will instinctively believe the brow tissue descending over the eyelid represents eyelid skin that can be removed. Browlifting in these cases can restore a more natural brow position but can also raise the pigment/cilia unnatural high, so this must be

Cleveland Clinic Foundation, Cole Eye Institute, 9500 Euclid Avenue, Cleveland, OH 44195, USA
* Corresponding author.
E-mail address: perryj1@ccf.org

Clin Plastic Surg 49 (2022) 409–414
https://doi.org/10.1016/j.cps.2022.03.002
0094-1298/22/© 2022 Elsevier Inc. All rights reserved.

discussed with the patient and considered in surgical planning.

Evaluation must include anatomic and patient factors. Anatomic factors include the brow height, position and contour, brow cilia density, forehead length, hairline position and thickness, and position and depth of forehead rhytids that could be used to conceal an incision.[5] For example, a patient with only 1 to 2 cm of distance from the lateral brow cilia to the lateral hairline would be a poor candidate for direct browlifting in this area, as it will bring the brow cilia unnaturally close to the lateral hairline. Patient factors include understanding their thoughts on the desired eyebrow contour and height, visibility of scars, length and location of possible visible scars, amount of acceptable downtime, and cost.[4] Choosing the technique for browlifting requires a careful balancing of all of these anatomic and patient factors.

The patient should be assessed for both dynamic and static brow asymmetry; the patient should be shown the difference between the 2 and instructed that lifting the brows only affects static brow position. Direct browlifting is often the most effective and predictable technique for addressing static brow position and in cases of unilateral brow ptosis. If the patient has one brow that is more dynamic than the other, neurotoxins may be required to improve this type of asymmetry, and the patient should understand this before surgery.

CONSIDERATIONS

Eyebrow ptosis occurs in older persons as a result of gravity and aging. Tissues of the forehead, eyelids, and upper face develop laxity with time, permitting the eyebrow to move inferiorly.[6] As a person ages, the normal, delicate attachments of the eyebrow to the periosteum become attenuated. As the eyebrow moves inferiorly, the frontalis muscle is recruited to elevate the eyebrow, which may result in deep horizontal forehead furrows. The lateral eyebrow lacks deep structural attachments to the periosteum and is especially susceptible to laxity.[7] Furthermore, the frontalis muscle fibers do not extend to the lateral brow, and thus, despite maximum frontalis contraction, lateral eyebrow ptosis often persists.[8] In severe cases, the lateral eyebrow may actually encroach on the eyelid space.

Patients with eyebrow ptosis may complain of dermatochalasis. However, when the eyebrows are raised to their normal position, there is often much less redundant upper eyelid skin than anticipated. Thus, assessing eyebrow position represents a critical aspect of upper blepharoplasty evaluation. Patients with eyebrow ptosis also show horizontal and vertical redundancy in the multicontoured areas of the medial and lateral canthi. These redundancies are a challenge for the aesthetic surgeon to correct through upper blepharoplasty alone.

It is important to remember that many factors participate in the aging of eyebrows and the forehead, not just brow position. Some of the brow descent and changes are due to volume loss, separation of the frontalis muscle from the orbicularis muscle laterally, and skin and bone changes. A higher brow is not always a more youthful brow. Indeed, raising the eyebrows in patients with previous aggressive upper blepharoplasty or in patients who have aged with loss of upper eyelid volume will unmask these aging changes. Unveiling a hollow upper eyelid can result in a more aged, skeletonized appearance and an unhappy patient, with few predictable options for improvement. The surgeon can use the mirror or digital imaging to show the patient potential outcomes and to understand the patient's aesthetic desires and concerns regarding the appearance of the upper eyelids as well as the brow position, height, and contour. With this information and by understanding the patient's goals regarding incision (scar) location and length, the surgeon can determine the type of browlift that will benefit the patient most.

Some cases of unilateral brow ptosis are due to seventh nerve paresis. In paralytic brow ptosis, because lagophthalmos is often present with many seventh nerve palsies, it is imperative that the brow not be overelevated, as this can worsen the lagophthalmos. The brow should generally be lifted in these cases only after the lagophthalmos has been minimized with eyelid weights or other techniques.

The choice of specific direct browlifting technique again depends on a variety of patient and anatomic factors relative to what the technique provides.[9] The supraciliary approach works best for patients with enough brow cilia to conceal the incision. This technique often leads to a nearly invisible scar laterally, so it can even be considered in some cases of lateral brow ptosis with even sparse lateral brow cilia. The placement of the incisions can allow for tailored contouring of the brows and works well for cases of preexisting brow asymmetry.[10] The midforehead approach works well for patients with deep forehead furrows. It can provide medial browlift for patients with central forehead fat pad ptosis. It can provide for lateral browlift if there is enough forehead between the brow and lateral hairline to allow for removal or for a pan-browlift if the patient is willing to accept longer scars and has a long forehead.

The frontalis transposition approach relies on transposition of the lateral extent of the frontalis muscle, to provide more elevated force to the lateral brow.[11] It works well for cases of mild to moderate lateral brow ptosis where a lateral horizontal rhytid is present within 1 to 2 cm of the superior brow cilia.

The transblepharoplasty, or internal browlift, relies on a glide plane created by the retro-orbicularis oculi and frontalis fat pad (ROOFF), part of the superficial musculoaponeurotic system.[8] It works for patients with mild amounts of lateral brow ptosis who do not want forehead scars, larger scalp incisions, or endoscopic approach. In the authors' experience it achieves only modest 1 to 2 mm brow elevation and is not suitable for patients with deep set eyes, hollow upper eyelids, or those with prominent ROOF tissue.

GOALS

Direct browlifting represents a compromise between the contour of the brow and the length and position of the resultant scar. Once that compromise has been determined preoperatively, the goal of surgery is to achieve the optimal height and contour of the brow, as determined by the patient, with minimal scarring and downtime and maximal predictability.

Once the decision has been made to consider a direct browlift, the next issue regards determining the location and length of the incisions; this will affect the brow contour. Some patients may rather have a smaller incision to treat only the lateral brow ptosis, whereas others may prefer a longer incision to achieve elevation for the entire brow. It is important to listen to the patient to understand their preferences.

The closer the incision is to the superior brow cilia, the more efficient the lift per millimeter of tissue excised. Some patients have rhytids in the midforehead that can be used to conceal the incision a bit. Some patients have only lateral brow ptosis and/or desire only lateral browlifting to limit

the length of the incision, and the lateral brow incisions generally heals much better than the medial brow incisions.

SURGICAL TECHNIQUE

All of the techniques for direct browlifting are very straightforward, and the procedures typically take less than 10 minutes per side. The techniques rely on basic anatomy. The main issues around direct browlifting regard the placement and length of the incisions.

Supraciliary Approach

With the patient in the sitting position, the proposed incision site is marked just above the most superior eyebrow hairs. The eyebrow is digitally elevated to the desired level, and the marking pen is placed near, but not touching, the superior brow border. When the brow is released, the point beneath the pen tip represents a point on the superior incision line. This marking technique is repeated along the entire incision line above the brow in the previously determined location for the incision. For example, if only lateral brow ptosis is evident, a segmental direct browlift can be performed.

The brow region is infiltrated with 2% lidocaine with 1 to 100,000 epinephrine solution containing hyaluronidase. The incision is carried out using a #15 Bard-Parker blade along the previously demarcated lines. The blade should be held perpendicular to the skin surface. In most cases, it is not necessary to bevel the incision, as some have suggested.

The depth of the incision is carried to a plane just superficial to the frontalis muscle in the region of the supraorbital neurovascular bundle to avoid bleeding and forehead hypesthesia. In patients with extreme lateral brow ptosis, the excised ellipse of tissue can extend more laterally than the lateral brow. However, the depth of the incision in the lateral portion is just through skin to avoid damage to the temporal branch of the seventh

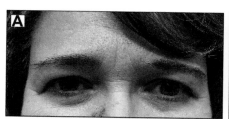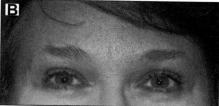

Fig. 1. Preoperative (*A*) and postoperative (*B*) appearance after a lateral supraciliary direct brow ptosis repair. The incision can hide well in this region. (Reprinted with permission, Cleveland Clinic Foundation ©2022. All Rights Reserved.)

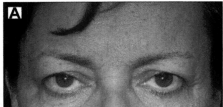 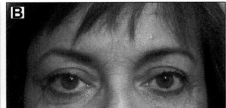

Fig. 2. Preoperative (*A*) and postoperative (*B*) appearance after a midforehead direct brow ptosis repair. This patient wears bangs and did not want to commit to cosmetically more concealed incisions and was pleased with the result. (Reprinted with permission, Cleveland Clinic Foundation ©2022. All Rights Reserved.)

nerve. In cases of paralytic brow ptosis, the frontalis muscle can be removed and the deep tissues suspended to the periosteum.

The ellipse of tissue is removed with scissors, a #15 blade, monopolar cautery, or radiofrequency device. The authors prefer the monopolar cautery in most cases. Hemostasis is achieved with monopolar and occasionally bipolar cautery.

The wound is closed with a deep layer of buried, interrupted 4-0 polyglactin 910 suture. The skin is closed with running 5-0 polypropylene suture. Some surgeons use multiple, interrupted vertical mattress sutures. The important consideration is eversion of the wound edge to avoid a depressed scar. The wound is dressed with antibiotic ointment, and ice compresses are applied 4 times a day for 2 to 3 days. The running superficial suture is removed in 7 days (**Fig. 1**).

Midforehead Approach

The skin is marked in much the same way as with the supraciliary approach, but using an existing forehead rhytid as the inferior margin of the incision. The incisions can be placed in rhytids of differing heights during bilateral surgery. Similar to the supraciliary approach, the skin and subcutaneous tissues are removed, preserving the frontalis muscle (**Fig. 2**).

Frontalis Transposition Approach

The incision is made along a lateral rhytid 1 to 1.5 cm in length, and subcutaneous dissection is performed to allow visualization of the fronto-orbicularis angle. This angle is created by the vertically oriented frontalis muscle fibers and the horizontally oriented orbicularis muscle fibers. A transposition flap of frontalis muscle is created with sharp dissection. This flap is then transposed laterally and trimmed to provide the optimal brow height. The frontalis muscle flap is then sutured to the orbicularis muscle with two 4-0 polyglactin 910 sutures. The skin is closed with running 5-0 polypropylene suture (**Fig. 3**).

Transblepharoplasty Approach

Through a standard upper blepharoplasty incision, sharp dissection is performed laterally within the deep ROOFF and above the periosteum approximately 2 cm above the orbital rim. Care should be taken to leave the periosteum and a small amount of very deep ROOFF tissue along and just above the orbital rim to prevent superficial adhesions to the orbital rim. This plane along the deep ROOFF is deep to the branches of the frontal branch of the facial nerve. The brow is then elevated to the desired height and the ROOFF tissues secured to the periosteum with a 4-0 polyglactin 910 suture in mattress fashion. The blepharoplasty incision is closed in standard fashion (**Fig. 4**).

POSTOPERATIVE THERAPEUTIC OPTIONS

It must be absolutely clear to the patient before surgery that direct browlifting leaves visible scars. The surgeon must ensure the patient understands and accepts this. Most patients heal well without need for further wound modulation. Indeed, scars along

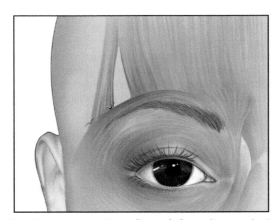

Fig. 3. A transposition flap of frontalis muscle is created to provide elevatory force to the lateral brow through a small incision concealed in a forehead rhytid. (Reprinted with permission, Cleveland Clinic Foundation ©2022. All Rights Reserved.)

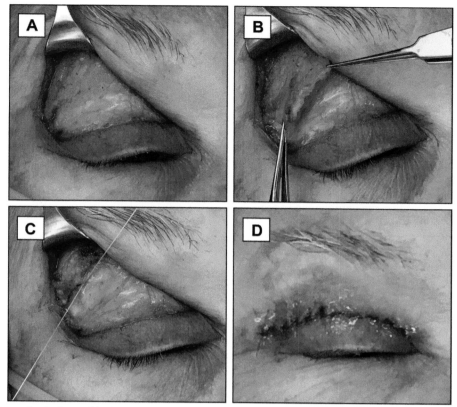

Fig. 4. This method of transblepharoplasty browlift uses a flap of retro-orbicularis oculi and frontalis muscle fat (ROOFF) that is trimmed (*A*), elevated (*B*), and secured (*C*) to the periosteum to buttress the lateral brow higher through a standard upper blepharoplasty incision (*D*). (Reprinted with permission, Cleveland Clinic Foundation ©2022. All Rights Reserved.)

the lateral supraciliary brow often heal nearly invisibly. Scars along the medial brow always heal thicker, and patients who are unwilling to compromise brow contour for scarring must accept this.

For thickened scars, various options are available to reduce the scar appearance. After 2 weeks, silicone scar gel can be used to try and decrease the scar. The silicone scar gel/sheets act as an occlusive dressing to help remodel the scar and decrease erythema and visibility of the hypertrophic scar. Intralesional injections of triamcinolone and/or 5-fluorouracil can be used after 4 to 6 weeks to help further remodel the scar. Dermabrasion or surface laser treatment can also be used to minimize the appearance of the scar.

Depressed scars are harder to treat. It is important to try to place incisions in an existing rhytid to conceal the scar. Deeply depressed scars can be treated with excision and resuturing.

FUTURE DIRECTIONS

Direct browlifting techniques continue to evolve as our understanding of the aging forehead anatomy improves. Minimal dissection involved with these techniques already satisfies one criterion of the ideal browlift. As our ability to modulate scarring improves and scars becomes less visible, these techniques will allow for optimal and predictable brow height and contour and will provide an increasing role in our armamentarium for the treatment of brow ptosis.

SUMMARY

Direct browlifting comprises powerful and efficient techniques to address brow ptosis. Scars are typically more visible than other techniques, but they can be minimized and modified.

CLINICS CARE POINTS

- Preoperative discussion with the patient is essential to decide with the patient where the visible scars will be.
- Incision location is based on patient tolerance for visible scar in the intended area and the amount, contour, and degree of browlift.

- Skin/subcutaneous tissue removal results in approximately a 1:1 ratio of brow elevation when the incision is in or at the brow.
- Frontalis muscle transposition lift can recruit elevatory force of the frontalis muscle laterally to improve lateral brow ptosis with a 1 to 1.5 cm incision along a midforehead rhytid.
- Trans-eyelid browlifting can improve mild lateral brow ptosis during upper blepharoplasty surgery.
- Scar modification with topical silicone gel application and intralesional 5- fluorouracil and steroid injection can improve the appearance of visible scars.

REFERENCES

1. Yalçınkaya E, Cingi C, Söken H, et al. Aesthetic analysis of the ideal eyebrow shape and position. Eur Arch Otorhinolaryngol 2016;273(2):305–10.
2. Hwang K, Yoo SK. Eyebrow shapes over the last century. J Craniofac Surg 2016;27(8):2181–4. PMID: 28005785.
3. Ridgway JM, Larrabee WF. Anatomy for blepharoplasty and brow-lift. Facial Plast Surg 2010;26(3): 177–85.
4. Kashkouli MB, Abdolalizadeh P, Abolfathzadeh N, et al. Periorbital facial rejuvenation; applied anatomy and pre-operative assessment. J Curr Ophthalmol 2017;29(3):154–68. Erratum in: J Curr Ophthalmol. 2018 Mar 06;30(2):188-189. PMID: 28913505;.
5. Chi JJ. Periorbital surgery: forehead, brow, and midface. Facial Plast Surg Clin North Am 2016;24(2): 107–17.
6. Knize DM. An anatomically based study of the mechanism of eyebrow ptosis. Plast Reconstr Surg 1996;97(7):1321–33.
7. Lemke BN, Stasior OG. The anatomy of eyebrow ptosis. Arch Ophthalmol 1982;100(6):981–6.
8. Blandford AD, Bachour SP, Chen R, et al. Dimensions and morphologic variability of the retro-orbicularis oculi and frontalis muscle fat pad. Ophthal Plast Reconstr Surg 2019;35(5):447–50.
9. Karimi N, Kashkouli MB, Sianati H, et al. Techniques of eyebrow lifting: a narrative review. J Ophthalmic Vis Res 2020;15(2):218–35.
10. Pelle-Ceravolo M, Angelini M, et al. Transcutaneous Brow Shaping: A Straightforward and Precise Method to Lift and Shape the Eyebrows. Aesthet Surg J 2017;37(8):863–75.
11. Ganapathy PS, Chundury RV, Perry JD. Safety and Effectiveness of a small incision lateral eyebrow ptosis Repair technique using a frontalis muscle transposition flap. Ophthalmic Plast Reconstr Surg 2016;32(6):438–40.

An Algorithm for Correction of the Aging Upper Face

James E. Zins, MD, FACS[a],*, Abigail Meyers, BS[b]

KEYWORDS

- Brow lift • Coronal brow lift • Minimally invasive • Endoscopic brow lift • Temporal brow lift
- Brow ptosis • Nonsurgical brow lift

KEY POINTS

- Brow lifting has evolved substantially over the past several decades with numerous less-invasive techniques largely supplanting the classic coronal brow lift.
- More recently, success in brow lifting is being measured not only by brow elevation alone but also by maintaining or improving brow shape.
- Endoscopic brow lifting and other less-invasive techniques have been popularized more recently, as well as nonsurgical options—each having specific indications and relative contraindications.
- Factors in the algorithm for choosing the ideal approach for each patient range from patient preference for technique invasiveness, brow shape, rhytid depth, hairline status, forehead length, and other considerations, such as age, gender, and medical comorbidities.

INTRODUCTION/BACKGROUND

The pertinent anatomy and ideal brow aesthetics have been addressed in detail in article one of this issue. A variety of brow-lift procedures have then been presented in the ensuing articles. In this article, the authors have attempted to put this wide variety of procedures into context with detailed indications and contraindications to each. Finally, an algorithm for choosing the proper brow-lift procedure is proposed.

APPROACHES TO CORRECTION OF THE AGING UPPER FACE
Open Techniques

Coronal brow lift
For the 30 years before the 1990s, the coronal brow lift was the mainstay for treatment of brow ptosis and forehead rhytids. Flowers and Ceydeli,[1] great proponents of the coronal lift, maintained that brow elevation alone would improve forehead rhytids by eliminating the need for constant

contraction of the frontalis muscle resulting from brow ptosis. In addition, they observed that by performing an upper-lid blepharoplasty in patients with brow ptosis, one can risk worsening the aesthetic result by removing the need for compensatory frontalis elevation. This may lead to an unsatisfactory result and worsening brow ptosis.

Despite long-term efficacy of the coronal lift, there are significant drawbacks that discourage its use. This includes potential for poor or widened scars, alopecia, and sensory loss. Because the deep branch of the supraorbital nerve runs between galea and periosteum just medial to the superior temporal line, it is more prone to injury during the coronal lift's subgaleal dissection (**Fig. 1**).[2–4] This can lead to chronic pruritis and other sensory changes. Although alopecia may occur temporarily in as many as 33% of coronal brow lifts, in many patients this resolves within 6 months.[5] Finally, patients often find the long scar a significant concern and therefore decline the procedure. Despite these drawbacks, the

[a] Section of Cosmetic Surgery, Department of Plastic Surgery, Cleveland Clinic, 9500 Euclid Avenue, Desk A60, Cleveland, OH 44195, USA; [b] Case Western Reserve School of Medicine
* Corresponding author.
E-mail address: zinsj@ccf.org

Clin Plastic Surg 49 (2022) 415–420
https://doi.org/10.1016/j.cps.2022.03.005

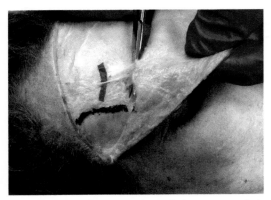

Fig. 1. Cadaver demonstration of the course of the deep branch of the supraorbital nerve. This branch passes 0.5 to 1.5 cm medial to the superior temporal line between periosteum and galea. It is therefore prone to injury during subgaleal dissection.

coronal brow lift remains the standard by which long-term efficacy of brow correction should be measured.

Coronal brow-lift indications:
- Significant brow ptosis
- Thick, sebaceous skin
- Deep forehead rhytids
- Normal or low forehead height

Coronal brow-lift relative contraindications:
- Thin or balding scalp
- Concerns regarding scarring
- Concerns for alopecia
- Minimal or isolated lateral brow ptosis

Endoscopic brow lift

The endoscopic brow lift introduced in the early 1990s appeared to avoid many of these drawbacks. It was touted as a minimally invasive technique with less scarring and a shorter recovery.[6–10] This initial enthusiasm was tempered when concerns regarding less-than-ideal results, early relapse, and other technical issues arose.[11] Specifically, overcorrection of the medial brow and lack of lateral brow elevation were common early findings. However, with increased experience, such problems have generally been overcome (**Figs. 2**A–D and **3**A–D). Medial brow elevation can be minimized by leaving at least 2 cm of periosteum attached at the glabellar midline. Lateral elevation is maximized by wide subperiosteal dissection, including the superior temporal line, the temporal ligamentous adhesion, and the lateral orbital rim extending down to the zygomatic arch. Wide subperiosteal undermining is generally considered more important than bone fixation. In fact, some question the need for any bone fixation.[12–14] Long-term studies by Jones and Lo[15] documented subtle, but persistent, correction of brow ptosis of just more than 4 mm at all points along the brow, except for the lateral-most point at the tail of the brow. This point reverted to its preoperative position 5 years after surgery.

Endoscopic brow-lift ideal candidates and surgical indications:
- Short or normal forehead height
- Flat forehead
- No true medial skin excess
- Nonreceding hairline
- Desire for small scars even with sparse hair
- Desire for minimally invasive procedure
- Minimal to moderate brow ptosis

Endoscopic brow lift: less than ideal candidates and relative contraindications:

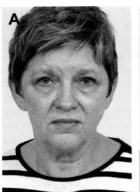 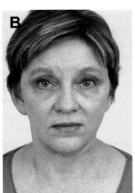 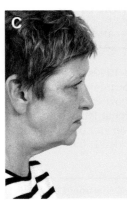 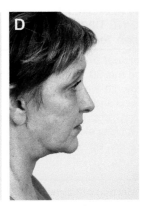

Fig. 2. (*A*) Preoperative frontal view of a 64-year-old woman who underwent extended SMAS facelift, subperiosteal endoscopic brow lift, and lower lid blepharoplasty. (*B*) Seven-month postoperative frontal view of patient seen in (*A*). (*C*) Preoperative profile view of patient seen in (*A*). (*D*) Postoperative profile view of patient seen in (*A*). SMAS; superficial musculo aponeurotic system.

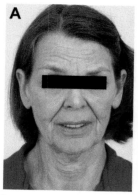 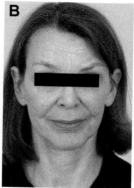 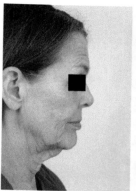 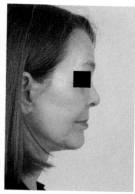

Fig. 3. (A) Preoperative frontal view of a 64-year-old woman who underwent deep plane facelift and endoscopic subperiosteal brow lift, perioral phenol croton oil peel, and fat grafting to the lower eye lids and malar region. (B) Postoperative frontal view of patient seen in (A). (C) Preoperative profile view of patient seen in (A). (D) Postoperative profile view of patient seen in (A).

- High or receding hairline
- Convex forehead
- Thick, sebaceous skin
- Deep frontalis lines
- True medial excess skin

Temporal brow lift

More recently, the importance of brow shape has been realized. Success in brow-lift surgery is not predicated on brow elevation alone. Eyebrow shape is perhaps even more important than brow elevation. This concept has been heralded in procedures, which address the lateral brow specifically, including the isolated temporal lift performed through a temporal hairline incision and the temporal lift performed through a limited lateral hairline incision, as described by Matarasso in article 4 of this issue.[16]

The isolated temporal hairline approach can be performed endoscopically[17,18] or under direct vision, as described by Knize and Spinelli.[19,20] This technique primarily addresses ptosis of the lateral third to half of the brow, the most common finding regarding the aging brow.[20,21] The dissection is taken down under direct vision to the deep temporal fascia, and then the dissection is extended onto the superficial layer of the deep temporal fascia medially to the lateral orbital rim. This is done with or without release of the superior temporal fusion line and the temporal ligamentous adhesion, depending on the severity of brow ptosis. This leads to correction of the loss of definition to the superior lateral orbital rim that occurs with aging. The isolated temporal lift as described by Matarasso includes a short hairline incision lateral to the midline, a subcutaneous forehead dissection, and an elliptical excision of forehead skin at the forehead-hairline junction. The isolated

temporal lift, when performed under direct vision, avoids the special equipment needs of the endoscopic approach. The medial brow depressor muscles, the corrugators, and procerus can also be treated at the time of temporal brow lifting by several ancillary means, including transpalpebral muscle resection, endoscopic resection, or botulinum toxin.

Temporal brow-lift indications:
- Need for isolated lateral brow elevation
- Short forehead
- Sparse hair
- Mild to moderate lateral ptosis

Temporal brow lift requires ancillary techniques to address the following:
- Need for medial brow elevation
- Need to modify corrugator muscles
- Deep rhytids

Hairline brow lift

The hairline brow lift, which involves a W-plasty–type incision the full length of the forehead-hairline junction, has noted a resurgence in recent years in part owing to the increased incidence of facial feminization surgery. The versatility of the hairline brow lift allows for both brow elevation and significant hairline lowering when a posterior subgaleal dissection is performed.[22,23] Relapse of brow lowering can be mediated using galeal scoring incisions parallel to the incision and cortical bone tunnels combined with progressive tension sutures (**Fig. 4**A–D).

Hairline brow-lift indications:
- High hairline
- Thin skin
- Thick hair
- Revision brow lifting

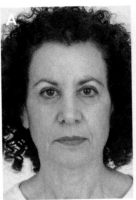 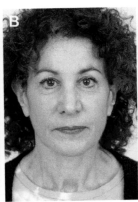 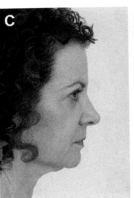 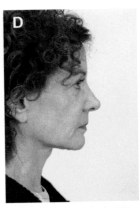

Fig. 4. (*A*) Preoperative frontal view of a 62-year-old woman who underwent extended SMAS facelift, hairline brow lift, and forehead-lowering procedure, including posterior subgaleal dissection, galeal scoring, and progressive tension sutures using cortical tunnels for fixation. (*B*) Three and a half years postoperative frontal view of patient seen in (*A*). (*C*) Preoperative profile view of patient seen in (*A*). (*D*) Postoperative profile view of patient seen in (*A*).

- Desire for facial feminization
- Desire to lower forehead height

Hairline brow-lift contraindications:
- Short forehead
- Receding hairline
- Significant brow asymmetry

Direct brow lift

Pelle-Ceravolo and colleagues in article 8 of this issue demonstrate that the direct brow lift does not need to be limited to elderly men. In a large patient series, Pelle-Ceravolo and Angelini[24] demonstrate outstanding results with minimal scars. Consistent with the current trend regarding brow shape, this operation allows for exacting brow-shape correction. The incision is tailored to the problem.[25,26] When lateral brow ptosis is all that requires correction, the incision can be limited medially, further minimizing the scar.

Direct brow-lift indications:
- Elderly men
- Medial brow elevation
- Selective tail elevation
- Unilateral brow ptosis
- Receded hairline
- Refuse major surgical procedures
- Compromised health, contraindications to general anesthesia

Direct brow-lift relative contraindications:
- Concerns regarding brow scar
- Short forehead
- History of hypertrophic scarring

Gliding brow lift

Exciting developments include newer techniques, such as a gliding brow lift, introduced by Viterbo

and colleagues[27] and recently popularized by Grotting. Grotting provides a detailed discussion and numerous preoperative and postoperative photographs in article 5 in this issue. The procedure is an extension of the hemostatic net.[28]

It avoids any significant scar entirely. A blind subcutaneous dissection is performed through small hairline stab incisions. Fixation is performed using transcutaneous sutures to first elevate the brow, and then additional running transcutaneous sutures are used to fix the forehead skin in place. Transcutaneous sutures remain in place for 48 hours only.

The benefit of scarless, minimally invasive surgery cannot be overstated, and Grotting's results are impressive. However, questions remain. This includes the questionable accuracy of the plane of dissection, the possibility of frontal branch injury if the subcutaneous plane is violated in the region of the frontal branch of the facial nerve, and the need for documentation of long-term efficacy.

Gliding brow-lift indications:
- Mild ptosis

Gliding brow-lift relative contraindications:
- Deep rhytids
- Thick sebaceous skin

Botulinum toxin injection

Finally, the chemical brow lift using botulinum toxin offers the possibility of subtle brow elevation as a minimally invasive office procedure.[29,30] Of course, the results are temporary and require reinjection on a 3- to 4-month basis. Botulinum toxin can also be used in combination with the isolated temporal lift to address corrugator muscle hyperactivity or as a subtle illustration of what can be

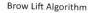

Brow Lift Algorithm

Fig. 5. The authors' algorithm for the correction of brow ptosis.

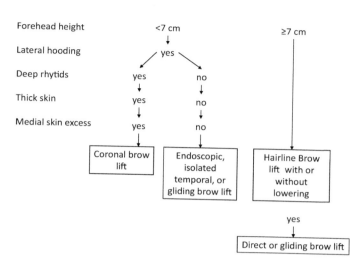

accomplished surgically. Similar to the endoscopic lift, the brow depressors are targeted and weakened, allowing the frontalis muscle to work relatively unopposed. Typically, the medial brow can be elevated approximately 1 mm, with the lateral brow lifting by as much as 4 mm.[31] Weakening of the frontalis muscle and improvement in horizontal lines can also be accomplished with botulinum toxin. However, this can exacerbate brow ptosis when toxin is used to treat frontalis lines lower on the forehead. Known injection complications include upper eyelid ptosis, exacerbation of brow ptosis, ecchymosis, and diplopia.[32]

Botulinum toxin indications:
- Desire for lateral brow elevation
- Desire for minimally invasive method

Botulinum toxin contraindications:
- Allergy
- Desire for more permanent effect

SUMMARY

In closing, the approach to brow lifting has changed perhaps more than any other facial aesthetic procedure in the past 20 years. Each surgical and nonsurgical approach has unique indications and relative contraindications Patient selection and preoperative assessment of the aforementioned characteristics, including rhytid severity, brow position, potential scarring patterns, surgical history, as well as patient expectations, should be assessed on an individual basis. The authors' algorithm for the correction of brow ptosis is detailed in **Fig. 5**. The authors hope this

issue and the guidelines discussed will provide a basis for enhanced surgical results and improved patient satisfaction.

CLINICS CARE POINTS

- Patients with thick, sebaceous skin, deep forehead rhytids, and significant brow ptosis seeking a relatively permanent solution may benefit most from a traditional coronal brow lift.

- The endoscopic brow lift and limited nonendoscopic variations of this procedure have in large part replaced the coronal brow lift because of the limited incisions and less-invasive nature of the procedure.

- The temporal brow-lift indications are ideal for lateral brow elevation in patients with sparse hair and only mild to moderate lateral ptosis. Ancillary techniques can be added to this procedure in order to address medial brow issues, including corrugator and procerus muscle hyperactivity or visibility.

- The hairline brow lift has had a resurgence owing to the recent popularity of facial feminization surgery. It can provide both correction of brow ptosis and forehead shortening.

- A direct brow lift has traditionally been reserved for elderly man with need for medial brow or selective tail elevation, unilateral brow ptosis (such as from facial nerve palsy), a receded hairline, and medical contraindications to general anesthesia. However, Pelle-Ceravolo and Angelini[24] have demonstrated excellent results in a wider range of patients.

- Botulinum toxin is a nonsurgical means of improving brow shape while providing subtle brow elevation on a temporary basis. It can also be used as a subtle illustration to the patient of what can be accomplished with surgical correction.

DISCLOSURE

The authors have nothing to disclose.

REFERENCES

1. Flowers RS, Ceydeli A. The open coronal approach to forehead rejuvenation. Clin Plast Surg 2008;35(3): 331–51.
2. De la Plaza R, Valiente E, Ma Arroyo J. Supraperiosteal lifting of the upper two thirds of the face. Br J Plast Surg 1991;4(5):325–32.
3. Tirkanits B, Daniel RK. The biplanar forehead lift. Aesthet Plast Surg 1990;14(1):111.
4. Ellenbogen R. Transcoronal eyebrow lift with concomitant upper blepharoplasty. Plast Reconstr Surg 1983;71(4):490–9.
5. Withey S, Waterhouse N, Witherow H. One hundred cases of endoscopic brow lift. Br J Plast Surg 2002; 55(1):20–4.
6. Aiache AE. Endoscopic face-lift. Aesthet Plast Surg 1994;18(3):275.
7. del Campo AF. Endoscopic forehead and face-lift: step by step. Open Tech Plast Reconstr Surg 1995;2(2):116–26.
8. Matarasso A, Terino EO. Forehead-brow rhytidoplasty: reassessing the goals. Plast Reconstr Surg 1994;93(7):1378.
9. Kashkouli MB, Beigi B. Endoscopy in the field of oculo-facial plastic surgery. J Curr Ophthalmol 2018;30(2):99–101.
10. Yeatts RP. Current concepts in brow lift surgery. Curr Opin Ophthalmol 1997;8(5):46–50.
11. Malata CM, Abood A. Experience with cortical tunnel fixation in endoscopic brow lift: the "bevel and slide" modification. Int J Surg 2009;7(6):510–5.
12. Guyuron B, Kopal C, Michelow BJ. Stability after endoscopic forehead surgery using single-point fascia fixation. Plast Reconstr Surg 2005;116(7): 1988–94.
13. Troilius C. Subperiosteal brow lifts without fixation. Plast Reconstr Surg 2004;114(6):1595–603.
14. Troilius C. A comparison between subgaleal and subperiosteal brow lifts. Plast Reconstr Surg 1999; 104(4):1079–90.
15. Jones BM, Lo SJ. The impact of endoscopic brow lift on eyebrow morphology, aesthetics, and longevity: objective and subjective measurements over a 5-year period. Plast Reconstr Surg 2013;132(2). https://doi.org/10.1097/PRS.0B013E3182958B9F.
16. Tabatabai N, Spinelli HM. Limited incision nonendoscopic brow lift. Plast Reconstr Surg 2007;119(5): 1563–70.
17. Savetsky IL, Matarasso A. Lateral temporal subcutaneous brow lift: clinical experience and systematic review of the literature. Plast Reconstr Surg Glob Open 2020;8(4). https://doi.org/10.1097/GOX. 0000000000002764.
18. Rohrich RJ, Cho MJ. Endoscopic temporal brow lift: surgical indications, technique, and 10-year outcome analysis. Plast Reconstr Surg 2019; 144(6):1305–10.
19. Eaves FF, Barton FE, Knize DM, et al. Comparative methods for brow lift. Aesthet Surg J 1997;17(6): 397–403.
20. Knize DM. Anatomic concepts for brow lift procedures. Plast Reconstr Surg 2009;124(6):2118–26.
21. Lemke BN, Stasior OG. The anatomy of eyebrow ptosis. Arch Ophthalmol 1982;100(6):981–6.
22. Dayan SH, Perkins SW, Vartanian AJ, et al. The forehead lift: endoscopic versus coronal approaches. Aesthet Plast Surg 2001;25(1):35–9.
23. Puig CM, LaFerriere KA. A retrospective comparison of open and endoscopic brow-lifts. Arch Facial Plast Surg 2002;4(4):221–5.
24. Pelle-Ceravolo M, Angelini M. Transcutaneous brow shaping: a straightforward and precise method to lift and shape the eyebrows. Aesthet Surg J 2017; 37(8):863–75.
25. Booth AJ, Murray A, Tyers AG. The direct brow lift: efficacy, complications, and patient satisfaction. Br J Ophthalmol 2004;88(5):688–91.
26. Green JP, Goldberg RA, Shorr N. Eyebrow ptosis. Int Ophthalmol Clin 1997;37(3):97–121.
27. Viterbo F, Auersvald A, O'Daniel TG. Gliding brow lift (GBL): a new concept. Aesthet Plast Surg 2019; 43(6):1536–46.
28. Auersvald A, Auersvald LA. Hemostatic net in rhytidoplasty: an efficient and safe method for preventing hematoma in 405 consecutive patients. Aesthet Plast Surg 2014;38(1):1–9.
29. Piovano L, D'Ettorre M. Forehead and brow rejuvenation: definition of a surgical algorithm. Eur J Plast Surg 2018;41(3):285–92.
30. Ilankovan V. Upper face rejuvenation. Int J Oral Maxillofac Surg 2013;42(4):423–31.
31. Kashkouli MB, Amani A, Jamshidian-Tehrani M, et al. Eighteen-point abobotulinum toxin a upper face rejuvenation: an eye plastic perspective on 845 subjects. Ophthal Plast Reconstr Surg 2014;30(3): 219–24.
32. Karimi N, Mohsen, Kashkouli B, et al. Techniques of eyebrow lifting: a narrative review. J Ophthalmic Vis Res 2020. https://doi.org/10.18502/jovr.v15i2.6740.

Moving?

Make sure your subscription moves with you!

To notify us of your new address, find your **Clinics Account Number** (located on your mailing label above your name), and contact customer service at:

Email: journalscustomerservice-usa@elsevier.com

800-654-2452 (subscribers in the U.S. & Canada)
314-447-8871 (subscribers outside of the U.S. & Canada)

Fax number: 314-447-8029

**Elsevier Health Sciences Division
Subscription Customer Service
3251 Riverport Lane
Maryland Heights, MO 63043**

ELSEVIER